Total Massage

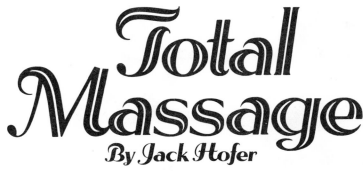

Total Massage

By Jack Hofer

Illustrated by Marjett C. Schille

Publishers · GROSSET & DUNLAP · New York
A FILMWAYS COMPANY

To Steve, Susan and Jacqueline; My father, Harold William Hofer, whose earthly touch suddenly ceased on January 25, 1952; My mother, Phyllis Rosetta Hofer, whose touch still abides.

Producing this work gave me an opportunity to focus my talents on the ever challenging task of bettering the human condition through the most important but neglected mode of communication—TOUCH.

From the start, my goal has been to make this the most readable, usable and enjoyable book of its kind ever published.

Jack Hofer

In my work, I try to help people to feel.

To me feelings of joy or sadness, enchantment or revulsion, tranquility or turbulence are equally valid. Each is a part of life.

The attempt to illustrate the sensations of pleasure, peace, sensuality and beauty inherent in massage was a challenging and fulfilling experience.

Marjett C. Schille

CONTENTS

FOREWORD

☐ I accepted with pleasure the task of writing a prefatory message for this book, because massage is one of the most ancient, effective means of obtaining relaxation from excessive stress in daily life.

☐ Although I know that Jack Hofer wishes to avoid as much as possible technical complexities, as the author of STRESS WITHOUT DISTRESS, I can not refrain from bringing up the point that, contrary to popular opinion, stress is not always harmful. It has been precisely the object of my latest studies to show how stress can be made to work for us, and what code of behavior is most conducive to the kind of stress that gives pleasure as well as a feeling of accomplishment and self-fulfillment. STRESS WITHOUT DISTRESS was designed to provide a natural code of conduct in life that would help us to avoid, as much as we can, "distress," or bad stress.

☐ However, since the medical concept of the stress mechanism and reactions to it has not yet been fully qualified, and because our capacity for the self-discipline needed to follow any code of behavior is limited, we shall always seek techniques that help us to reduce distress and to relax. This is true, no matter how highly developed our behavior is, no matter what final goals we pursue in life.

□ Not only can massage help to reduce distress, it can be effective in producing favorable stress, "eustress" (eu = good, as in euphoria, euphonia). Although the general public is less familiar with this concept, scientists acknowledge that there is such a thing as pleasant stress. If we define stress as "any demand made upon the body," we can readily see that some demands would be positive, others negative.

□ In addition to the various psychologic techniques aimed at relaxation, such as transcendental meditation, Jacobson's progressive relaxation technique, yoga, and Zen, physical procedures, in the form of sports, hydrotherapy, and acupuncture, among others, have always enjoyed great popularity. Massage is certainly a very important member of this latter group.

□ Aided by beautiful drawings depicting a step-by-step approach to the art of massage and the pleasure it can give, Jack Hofer's book will greatly benefit the many people who are in need of it.

Hans Selye
M.D., Ph.D.
Professor and Director
Institute of Experimental Medicine and Surgery
University of Montreal
Montreal, Canada

INTRODUCTION

It is clear that the decisive form of our
intercourse with things is in fact touch.
And if this is so, touch and contact are
necessarily the most conclusive factor
in determining the structure of our world.
                                        Ortega y Gasset

The modern world is a complex place to live. Conse-
quently, people become anxious, uptight and out of touch
with themselves and others around them. In this book I
am going to bring you back to the instinct of touching as
a means of communicating a sense of relaxed and warm
feelings toward yourself and others.

□ A simple, direct and successful approach to accom-
plishing this mellow state is a total body massage. I'm
speaking of an everyday type of massage that everyone
can learn to do. Massage, or what can be referred to as
SKILLED TOUCHING, is a technique for revitalizing the
mind and body. With practice, it always yields positive
results by increasing circulation, sensation, energy and
a sense of well-being. It reduces stress, produces relaxation, promotes restful sleep and develops a bond between
people. Massage feels good and costs nothing. It can be
done in a variety of places: at home or at a friend's place,
on the beach, in a park or even in a field of wild flowers,
if there happens to be one handy.

□ The word MASSAGE frequently raises negative asso-
ciations in peoples' minds. My intentions are to take the
word out of the context of "sleezy massage parlors" and
"sterile clinics" and put it in its rightful place in the
spectrum of heightening human awareness.

□ Touching and massaging are forms of communication
without words. During a massage, a feeling of caring is
relayed from the giver to the receiver. Recent psychological studies have shown that giving and receiving affection account for more than 70 percent of the ten most
important and enjoyable activities in a person's life. Affection is defined here as a secure, kind and loving feeling directed toward others or received from others.

12

☐ A gentle, soothing massage can bring family members, friends or lovers closer together. If practiced regularly within a family, children and parents will come into a closer relationship than could ever be possible through the use of words, money and material objects. When we were children we gave and received lots of personal loving body contacts. As we grew up and "matured," we strayed from touching behavior, not realizing how vitally important it is for human contentment and fulfillment. In some countries, particularly in Europe, people tend to touch each other several times during the course of a conversation. In the United States, however, many people rarely, if ever, touch one another.

☐ As Desmond Morris, author of INTIMATE BEHAVIOR, reveals, "Something special happens when two people touch each other. The soothing and calming effects of gentle intimacies leave the individual freer and better equipped emotionally to deal with the more remote, impersonal moments of life. They do not soften him as has so often been claimed; they strengthen him."

☐ You've probably heard the saying, "A picture is worth a thousand words." In designing and writing this book, I have carefully chosen the word/picture combinations to allow you to learn massage in an easy, pleasant, uncomplicated manner. Instructions have been kept to a minimum to eliminate unnecessary and tiresome reading. Only enough information has been presented to help you keep things flowing smoothly. The idea was to combine only the essential words with pleasant and informative illustrations that accurately depict the art of massage.

☐ I have avoided highly technical, clinical and anatomical descriptive information. Instead, you will find familiar, everyday analogies, spiced with a bit of humor. Massage is not only soothing and relaxing, it is also fun. It is not a science, so you don't have to be all that precise. All you need is some initial guidance, a little practice, and soon you will be flying high.

☐ How do you use this book? First, look through it from cover to cover. Scan through the text if you feel like it. Then read Section 1, PRELIMINARIES. Next, take some time and thoroughly read Section 2, A TOTAL BODY MASSAGE. This is the most important section in the book. It will provide you with the basic skills for delivering a superb massage. You can prop the book up against a piece of furniture or some other sturdy object if you are giving a massage to a person lying on the floor, or, on a table or stand if you are massaging someone on a massage table. Body contact at all times is important to keep the energy and relaxation flowing, so keep one hand on your partner while using the other hand to turn the page.

☐ Don't worry about remembering every movement exactly. You will develop your own techniques as you go along since everyone giving or receiving a massage has his or her own personal preferences. Let your partner be your guide. The main consideration is to make your partner comfortable and happy. Once you have practiced a total body massage a few times, turn to whatever section interests you: massaging yourself or a child or performing an erotic or group massage. Do whatever comes naturally, as long as you do not cause the person receiving the massage any discomfort.

☐ Section 4, MASSAGING YOURSELF, shows how to give an acceptable massage to yourself. The latter part of

Section 4 is a kind of home remedy kit on how to relieve five of the most common body aches and complaints.

☐ Section 7, OTHER CONSIDERATIONS, contains information on stress, diet, weight control, exercise, natural breathing and posture. In addition, ways of relaxing such as yoga and meditation are presented along with other information essential to health and happiness.

☐ Massage is a nonverbal bond between giver and receiver. It has many beneficial physical effects, but the most important are the personal ones. A bit of practice and caring will soon identify you as a LIFETIME DISPENSER OF MIND-BODY PLEASURE.

ONE
PRELIMINARIES

Happiness is the only good
The time to be happy is now
The place to be happy is here
The way to be happy is to make others so.
Robert Green Ingersoll

The word MASSAGE comes from the French verbs MACER or MASSER. These words were first used in 1779 by a French adventurer named Le Gentil when he wrote a book entitled VOYAGE ON THE INDIAN OCEAN.

FORMS OF MASSAGE

There are over fourteen different forms of massage:

French	Esalen
Swedish	Reichian
German	Polarity Therapy
Oriental	Zone Therapy
Cosmetic	Reflexology
Proskauer	Acupressure
Shiatsu	Remedial Gymnastics

☐ Many of these massage techniques involve movements that are used primarily in physical therapy. The massage form presented in this book includes several features adapted from these forms, plus many of my own techniques. You will not become a physical therapist by reading this book, but you will learn a proven method for giving a soothing and relaxing massage. As a result, many physical problems will disappear as unnecessary tension and stress are relieved.

☐ The above forms of massage involve several thousand movements. You don't have to know many different movements in order to deliver a good massage. All you need to know are a few basic movements to apply to various areas of the body. In this book you will be given ten basic movements.

Anatomy and physiology are complex and boring subjects. You really don't need to know much about either one to use the techniques presented in this book. If after you have used these techniques you feel that knowing more about muscle, bone and skin structure will help you to give a better massage, then refer to any textbook on those subjects.

☐ Here, however, are a few things that you do need to know:

SOME ANATOMY AND PHYSIOLOGY

Muscles are connected to bones.

☐ When muscles contract they are in a state of tension. When muscles lengthen or become loose, they are in a state of relaxation.

Muscles

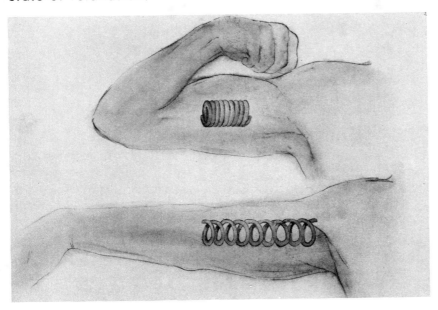

Throughout the course of giving massages you will learn, mostly by touch, when a muscle is in a state of tension and when it is in the pleasant realm of relaxation. You will spend more time on those areas of the body that are tense and less time on those areas that are not uptight.

Bones There is no need for you to learn the formal names of the many bones in the human body. All you need to know is that bones will break or become injured if subjected to too much pressure or movement.
☐ No dangers are involved when you employ proper applications of the techniques presented in this book. I am teaching you the art and skill of giving a GENTLE and RELAXING massage.

Joints Joints are where two bones come together. They are not to be moved beyond COMFORTABLE limits.
☐ Do not massage or move a joint that has been injured or sprained.

Skin and Blood Vessels The human skin contains over half a million sensory nerve endings. The sensors of heat, cold and pain account for about half of the nerve endings and touch receptors comprise the rest. These touch receptors are in our bodies for a purpose—to be touched.
☐ The human skin and blood vessels are amazingly flexible and pliable. They can, however, become injured if too much pressure, pulling or pounding occurs during a massage. GENTLE but firm movements will prevent bruising

or injuring the skin and blood vessels. Using oil will reduce friction.

☐ Do not massage skin that has an open sore, cut, bruise, burn or other injury.

The human body is a well-regulated heat factory kept at about 98.6° Fahrenheit.

☐ If the temperature of the body drops even a small amount, the person will become CHILLED and SHIVERING will set in, muscles will become TENSE and you will have blown the whole massage.

☐ The room temperature should be about 75°. Use a sheet, if necessary, to keep the person comfortable while being massaged.

Body Temperature

The human body is POETRY IN MOTION when it is relaxed and functioning properly. It can become a LOADED GUN when wracked by nervous tension, stress and anxiety.

☐ To unwind the body and mind, a person first has to be put at ease. Whether or not someone is put at ease depends on how you approach the person, what you say, the setting of the massage and the initial preparation. All of these will be discussed in a moment.

☐ Here are some essential hints when giving a massage:

Body Dynamics

- most folks will gladly volunteer for the benefits of a good massage.
- if, however, someone is uptight, try to convince him or her to try massage once. After that, most people become believers.

21

- once your partner is lying down with eyes closed, half the battle is over.
- massage is a direct form of nonverbal communication.
- concentrate totally on the massage and the person being massaged.
- find out from the person you will be massaging if there are specific tensions and, if so, spend more time working on those areas.
- you will gradually learn to feel out and relieve tenseness in muscles and connective tissue.
- massage can have a stimulating and invigorating effect as well as a relaxing and sedative effect.
- use gentle-to-firm movements.
- avoid working on very painful areas of the body.
- keep the body warm at all times.
- if your partner gets the tickles, move to another area and try coming back later on (sometimes heavier pressure gets rid of the tickles).
- be aware of the flow, rhythm and exchange of energy.
- massage will heighten your sense of touch so that you will become more aware of the texture and substance of everything you come into physical contact with.
- let the person receiving the massage be your guide to a pleasant, energy-exchanging experience.

SETTING The setting can have a lot to do with the success of your massage. The room or place of massage should be:

22

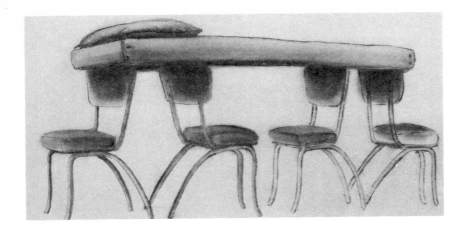

- free from distractions (ringing telephone) or other disturbances.
- free from direct or harsh lighting (try using a low-wattage green or blue light bulb).
- warm and comfortable.

A massage can be given on a table (if the size is correct) or on the floor. Do not give someone a massage on a BED. (The exception is when giving an erotic massage since there you will be limiting the number of movements to a few areas that lend themselves to being massaged and stroked while the person is lying on a bed.) A total body massage on a bed may feel great to the person receiving it but it results in unnecessary strain and fatigue for the person giving it.

☐ If you happen to have a sturdy table about 6 feet long, 2 feet wide and 32 inches high, then you are in business. Foam padding, blankets or soft material can be used on top of the table.

☐ If you don't have a table, you can make one that will store upright in a closet or under a bed. Take a piece of plywood or composition board that measures six feet by two feet. Using 1-by-4-inch pine, some nails and glue, build some sides and ends on your table. Then place four sturdy kitchen chairs with flat tops evenly under the table and you will be in business.

☐ The seats of the two end chairs should stick out from the table so you can sit down while working on the head or feet. Cover your table with foam, cloth, leather, vinyl, fur or whatever turns you on.

☐ If you have the room for a permanent massage table,

23

you can add sturdy legs to your table by bolting six legs made of 4-by-4 pine to the ends and center. Then place pieces of 1-by-4 pine along the sides and at the ends, about halfway down the legs, to make the table more secure.

☐ If you want a massage table but do not wish to build your own, you may receive information on quality folding or permanent massage tables by writing to the address listed on page 222.

☐ If you don't have a table, then the floor is the answer. Even with carpeting you will need a foam pad (about 4-by-8 feet), a couple of blankets or a folded-out sleeping bag. If you are outdoors, a blanket on top of the grass, sand or a field of wild flowers will suit the purpose very nicely.

Music

The right kind of music can enhance a massage. The best kinds seem to be light classical and soft background music.

☐ A couple of my favorite albums are:

- Sound track for the movie JONATHAN LIVINGSTON SEAGULL, by Neil Diamond (Columbia).
- MAESTRO SEGOVIA, by Andrés Segovia (Decca).

☐ Music has to have the right rhythm and flow. Keep the volume low and at a pleasant level. It is far better to have no music at all than to play fast-moving lively selections.

Room Temperature

Keep the room at approximately 75°.

☐ You can wrap a sheet or blanket around the person's

24

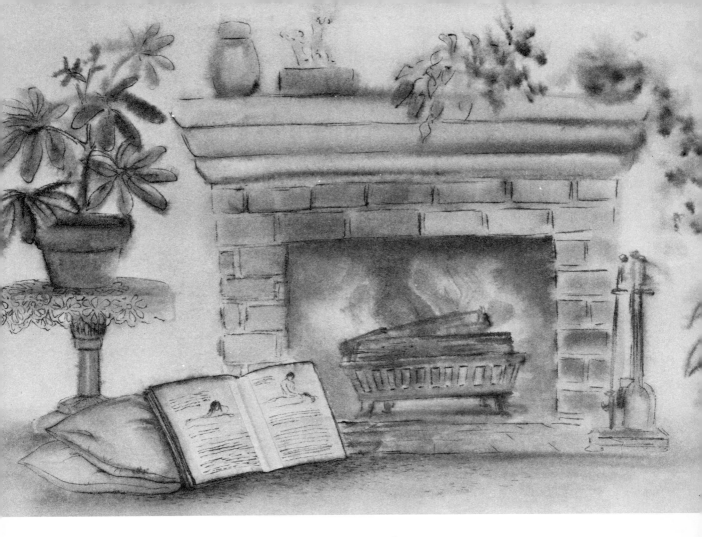

body to cover those areas you are not massaging at the moment. A heat lamp may be used but keep it at a safe and comfortable distance from the body.

☐ Do not use a hair dryer or any other kind of electrical appliance to warm the body.

Oils

Oil helps reduce skin-surface tension and friction. Use only oils that you can take internally. This means for the most part vegetable, fruit or nut oils. Try to use the lightest oil possible. The best thickness for oil is a viscosity slightly heavier than water.

☐ Use only a few drops of oil for each area. Always apply a few drops to the palm of your hands and rub them together before placing your hands on the person's body. A little more oil will be necessary on hairy parts of the body. Do not use too much oil.

25

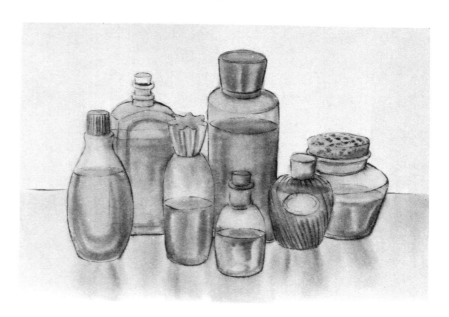

☐ Experiment and find one or two oils that you like. You can add a few drops of your favorite perfume or scent to the oil: mint, eucalyptus, clove, pine, orange, lemon, lime, strawberry, anise, vanilla, almond, musk, etc. You may want to heat the oil in a container placed on top of a food warmer or room heater.

☐ Your skin is a very important part of your body so treat it well. Avoid using mineral, baby oil or petroleum-based oils or hand lotions whenever possible, as synthetic oils are greasy and will clog the pores. If you use lotions, make sure they are made from natural ingredients.

FASHION Clothing is out. Birthday suits are in.

☐ Some people may be uptight about removing all of their clothing for the first massage. Later on this is usually not a problem. If someone feels uncomfortable with complete nudity, suggest that panties, shorts or a bathing suit be worn. The LESS clothing involved the BETTER the massage.

26

A 5- or 10-minute warm bath, shower or sauna serves to cleanse the skin, open pores and increase circulation. This, coupled with a brisk rubdown with a thick towel and having the person wrap a large dry towel around the body, is a good method of putting the person at ease. Later on the towel can be removed and replaced with a sheet.

☐ Do not massage a person until one hour after a meal or strenuous exercise.

PREPARATION

An electrical vibrator may be used on the back of the neck and shoulders and on the arms, thighs, calves, buttocks and bottoms of the feet. DO NOT USE it on the face, front of neck, ribs, knees, elbows, shins, spine or abdominal area.

☐ Other accessories of pleasure are a large feather, a piece of fur or a lightweight silk scarf. You will be told what to do with these later on.

ACCESSORIES

Make sure the person receiving the massage removes glasses or contact lenses.

☐ Ask the person to lie down with back on the massage table or floor pad. Have the person close both eyes and breathe deeply.

☐ Be considerate and don't push or rush anything before, during or after a massage.

A FINAL SUGGESTION

27

TWO
A TOTAL BODY MASSAGE

If only all the hands that reach, could touch.

Loberg

This is the most important section in the book. Here is where you will learn the essential movements for giving a soothing and relaxing massage.

THE TEN BASIC MASSAGE MOVEMENTS

Learn these ten basic movements well. They will be applied to different areas of the body.

effluerage

(Pronounced Ef-luh-rahj)
☐ Long light gliding strokes made with the entire inside surface of the hands.
☐ Used on: arms, legs, back and chest.

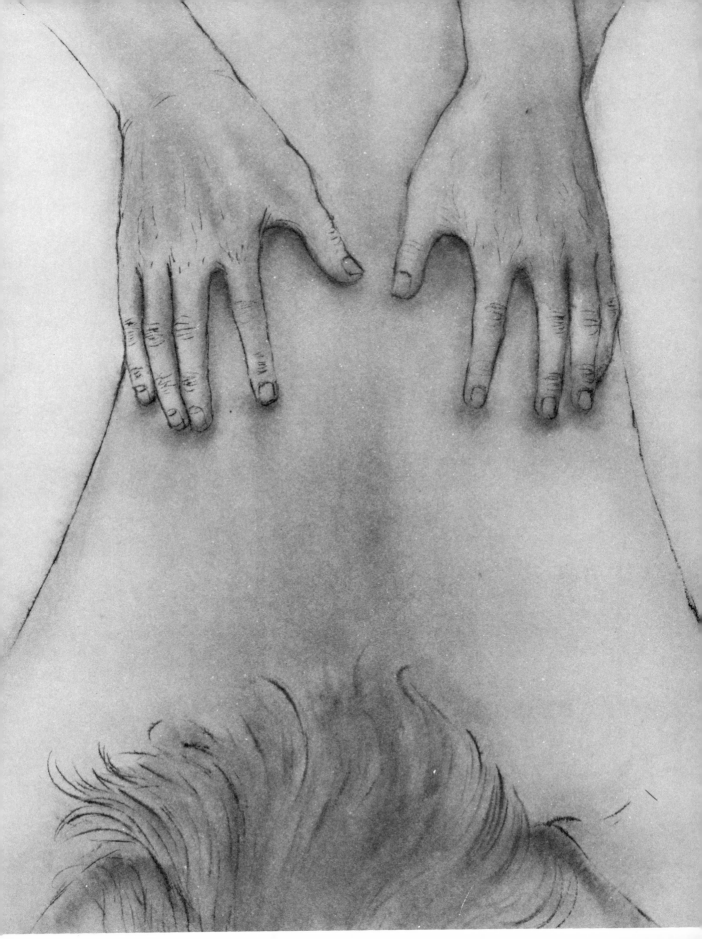

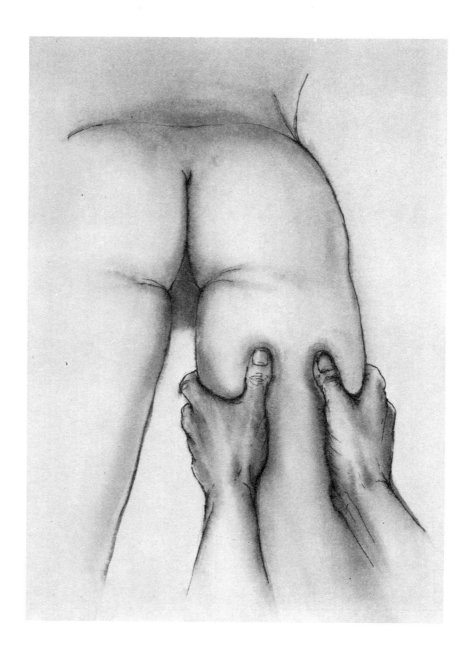

kneading Firm grasping pressure used to move muscles and skin. It is like kneading flour dough to make bread.
☐ Used on: abdominal region, buttocks, arms, legs, hands and feet.

32

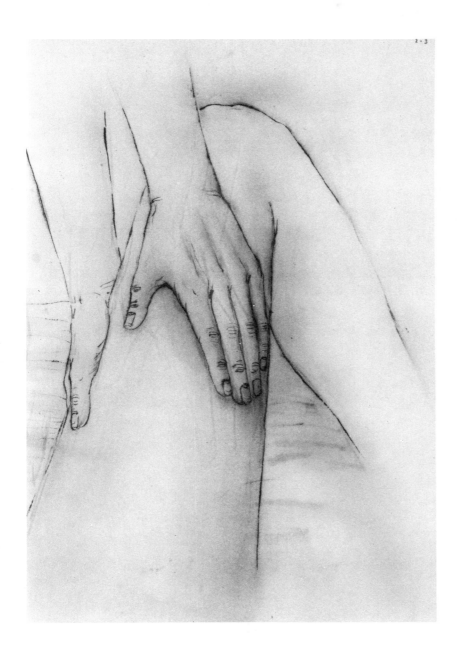

Used for moving large skin masses. It is like rolling clay **rolling**
between your hands.
☐ Used on: thighs, calves of legs, upper arms and buttocks.

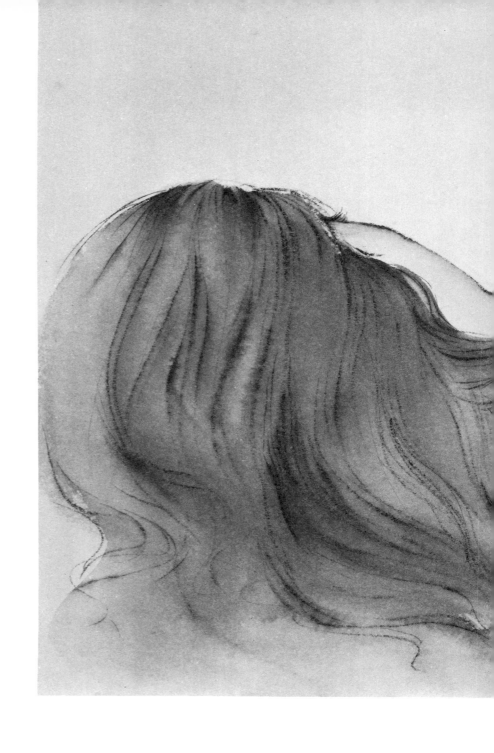

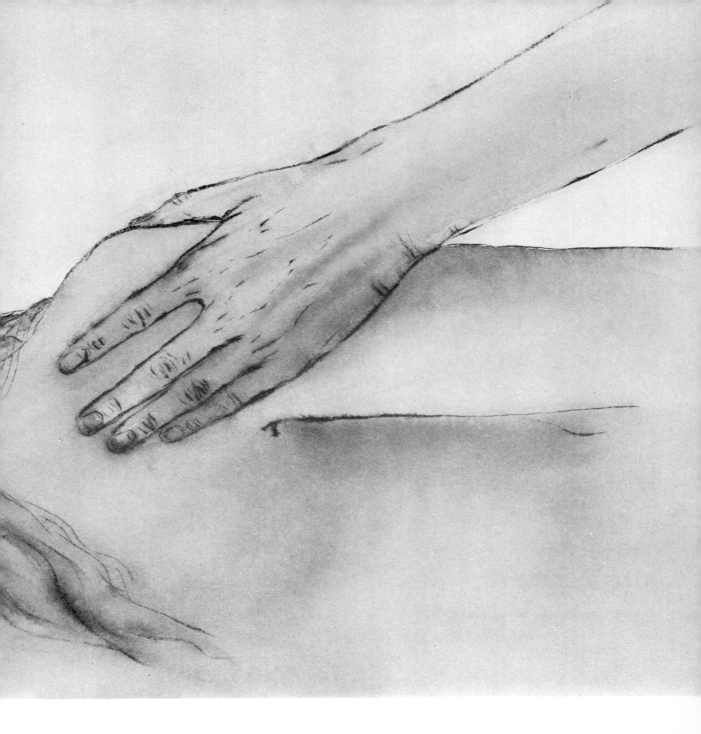

Gentle movements of the joints. The movements should **rotation**
be loose, not forced.
☐ Used on: shoulder/arm, wrist, ankle, neck, elbow and
knee joints.

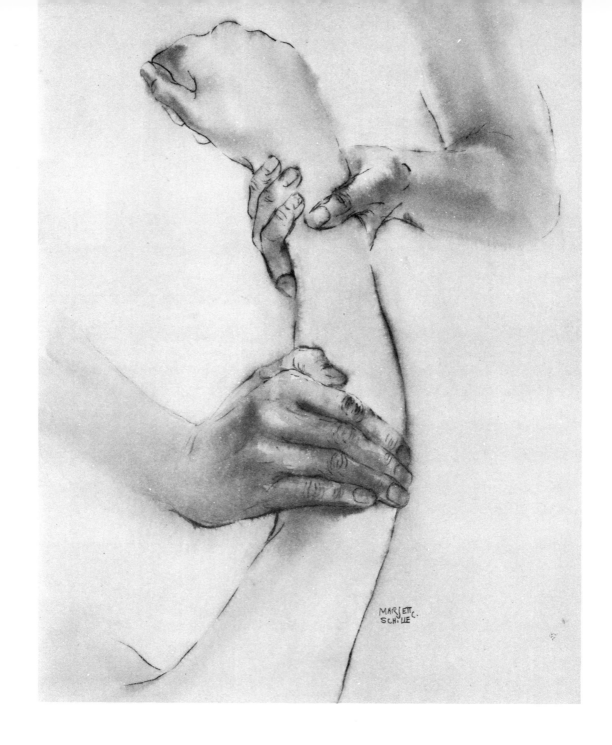

friction   Two types:

      1. Long, slow and firm stroking movements. Used on: back, chest, arms and legs.

36

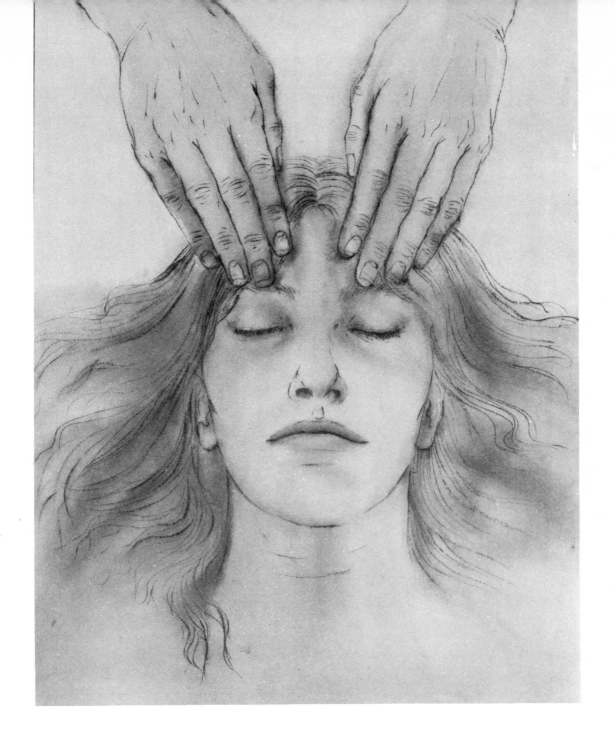

2. Small, circular movements using the tips of your fingers, balls of your thumbs, and heels of your hands. Used on: head, neck, elbow, knee and ankles.

petrissage   (Pronounced Pet-rah-sahj)....

☐ Picking up skin between the thumb and fingers, squeezing the skin gently and dropping it back into place. It is like gently pinching the skin of a furry cat.

☐ Used on: back, underside of upper arms, and backs of the legs.

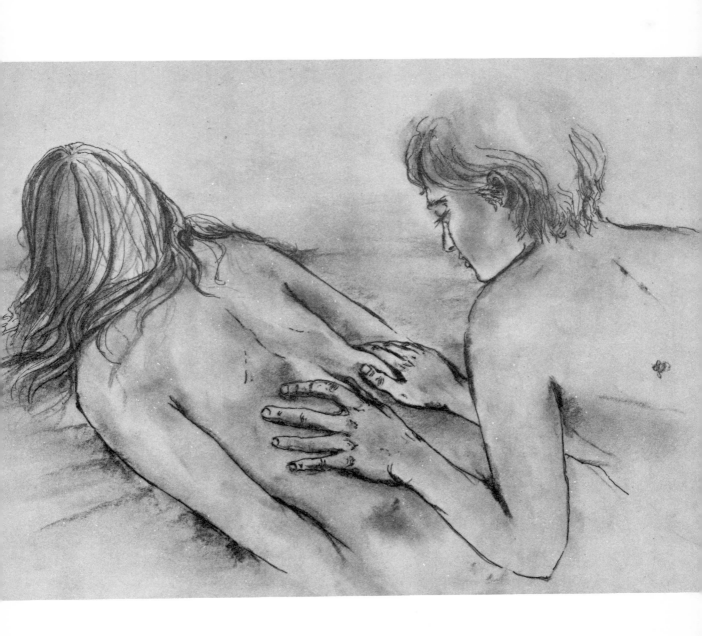

pressure pull Firm, constant pulling pressure.
□ Used on: Entire back, also top of the hand to tips of fingers and top of thigh to tips of the toes (one direction only).

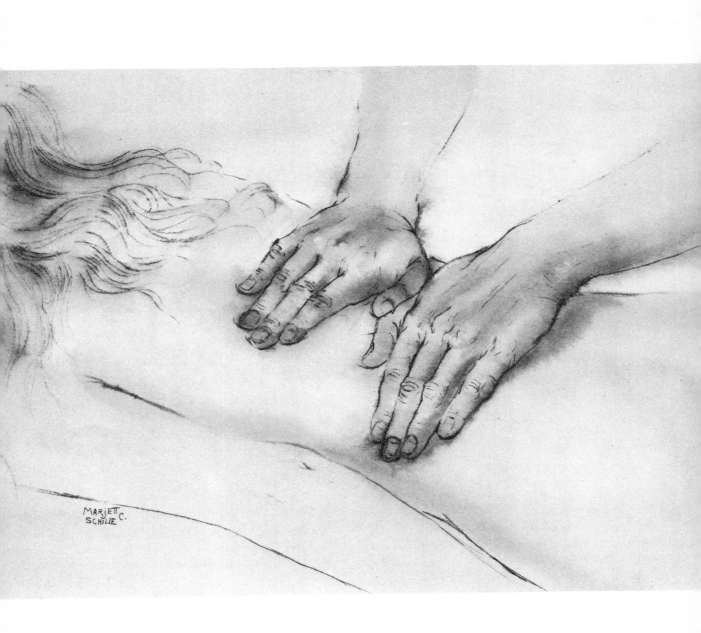

vibration Very rapid back-and-forth shaking movements made with both hands. It is like shaking a bowl of Jell-O.
□ Used on: upper back, buttocks and thighs.

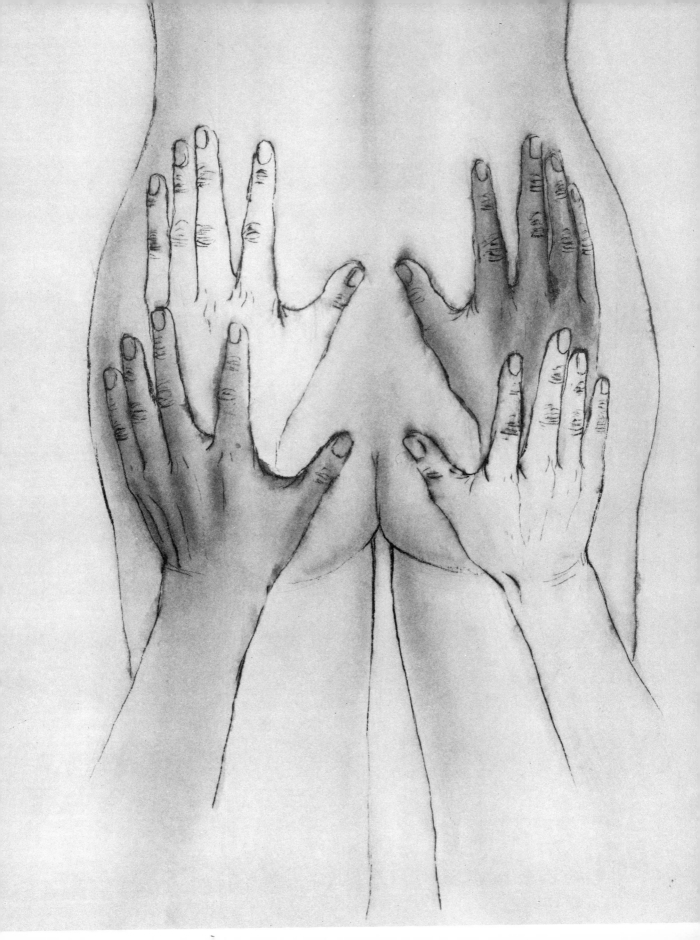

Percussion Movements:
tapping
hacking
cupping
slapping

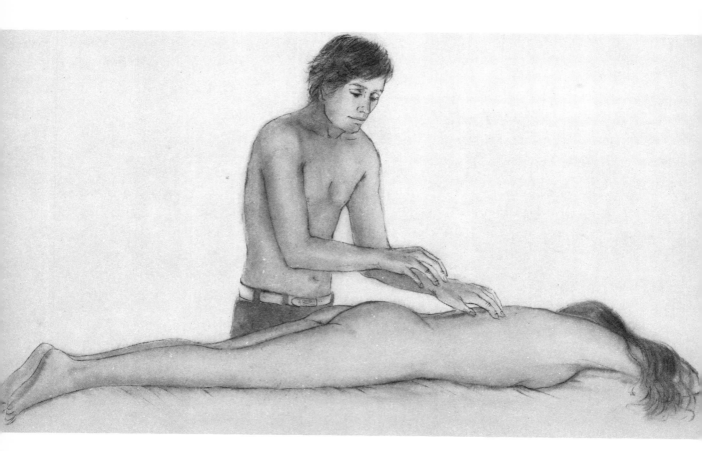

tapping ☐ Rapid alternate movements of fingertips striking the body.

☐ Spread the fingertips of both hands into the shape of a garden rake. When you are doing this movement properly, you should feel and hear a kind of DULL thump-thump sound.

☐ Used on: Entire back surface of the body.

☐ Used to: Stimulate nerve endings.

44

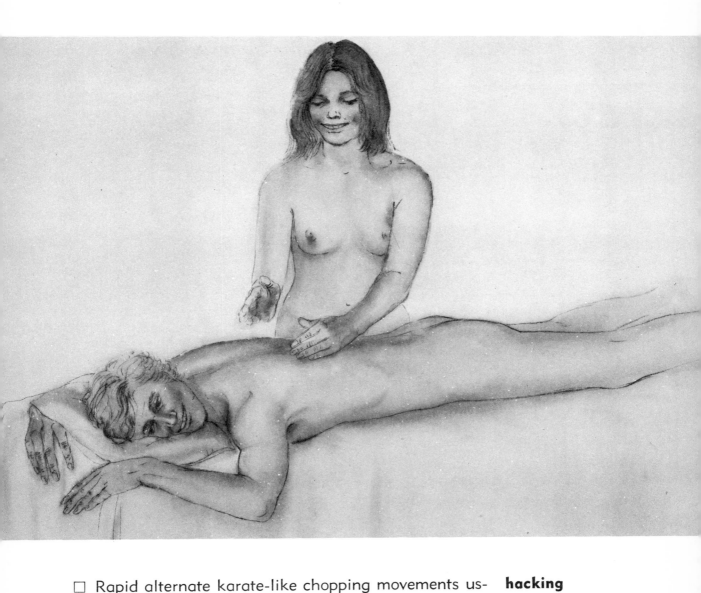

☐ Rapid alternate karate-like chopping movements us- **hacking**
ing both hands.

☐ Make the hands into the shape of a knife. When you
are doing this movement properly, you should feel and
hear a kind of FLAT clump-clump sound.

☐ Believe me, this feels a lot better than it sounds.

☐ Used on: Entire back surface of the body.

☐ Used to: Increase circulation.

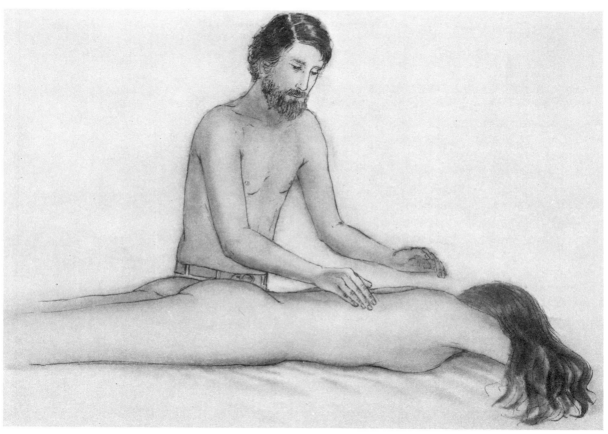

cupping ☐ Rapid alternate cupped-hand movements made with both hands.
☐ Make your hands into the shape of a cup or seashell. Go clop-clopping all over the entire back surface of the body. When you are doing this movement properly, you should feel and hear a HOLLOW whop-whop sound.
☐ Used on: Entire back surface of the body.
☐ Used to: Relax muscles.

46

☐ Rapid alternate slapping movements made with both **slapping** hands.
☐ Make your hands flat like a pancake. When you are doing this movement properly, you should feel and hear a slightly SHARP smack-smack sound.
☐ Used on: Entire back surface of the body.
☐ Used to: Heighten skin sensations.

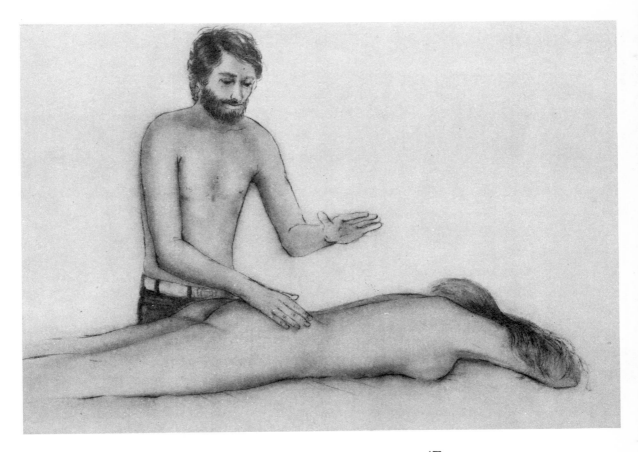

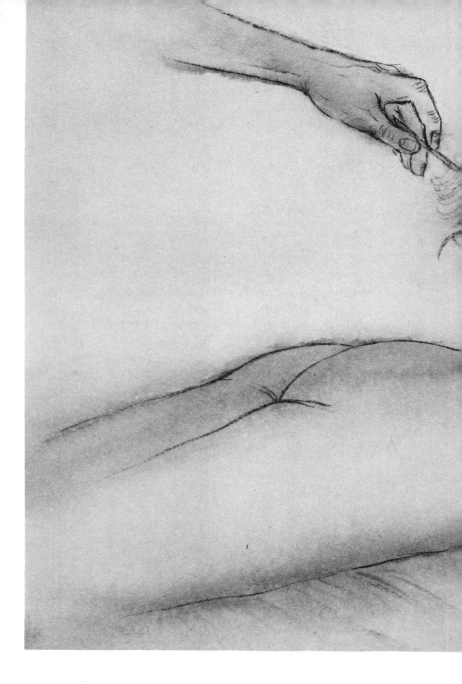

feathering Light dragging movements made with both hands or another object.
  □ Made by dragging fingertips or large feather or silk scarf or piece of fur or anything that feels good over the body.
  □ Used on: Entire back surface of the body.
  □ Used to: Put icing on the cake.

48

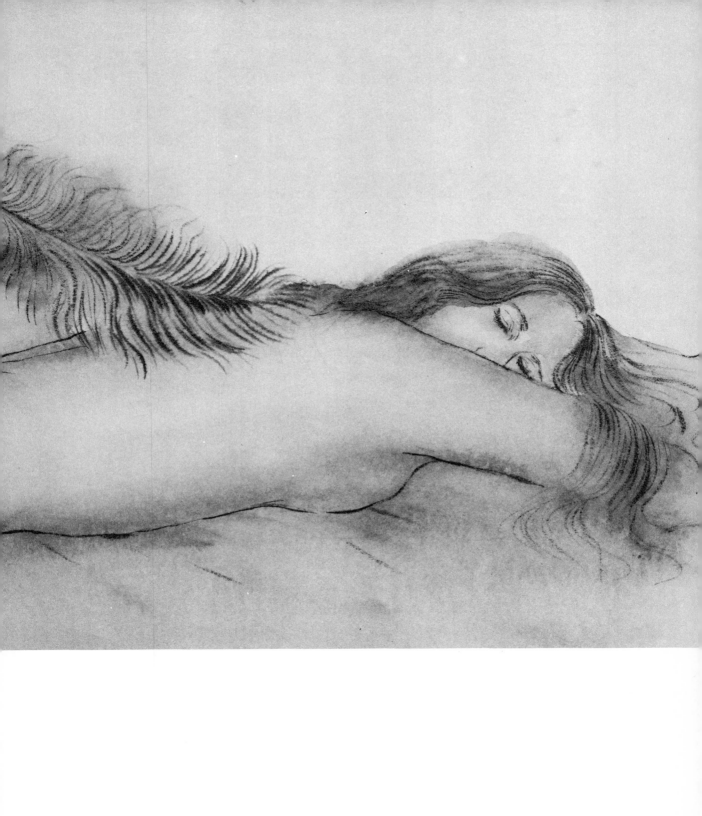

THE TOTAL BODY MASSAGE

Now you are ready to dispense some pleasant relaxation.
☐ Take plenty of time. Never rush through a massage. If time is a factor, do only two or three areas. Or, use light strokes over the entire body.
☐ Do not attempt to give a Total Body Massage if you are overly tired. It is better to spend only a few minutes on one or two areas of the body and wait until you are rested and relaxed before attempting a full body massage.
☐ In a Total Body Massage you are approaching the body as one balanced and complete system. Let your hands and partner be your guide.
☐ Here are a few things to remember the first few times you give a massage:

- it may take a little time for a person to get used to the feel of YOUR hands on his or her body.
- as you get into the massage, your partner will loosen up and relax.
- body and mind will let go and unwind like a peaceful river wandering on its way to an ocean of pleasure.
- after a few times you will become surprisingly adept at giving a soothing massage.
- most people will be very responsive to a gentle, stimulating, caring massage since it is direct contact with the body, skin and nervous system.

☐ When giving a massage, get into the FEEL and RHYTHM of your partner's body. Maintain a nice, even rhythm.

50

☐ Ask the person to lie down on the back, close the eyes and do deep, natural breathing.

☐ If a person has been particularly tense for a long period of time, then it may take a few massages to really loosen up those tight, held-in feelings.

☐ When first learning, practice on one or two areas of the body at a time. After you feel confident about your ability to pleasure those areas, move on to a couple more areas of the body. Finally, put them all together and practice the entire body massage.

☐ Never massage one arm or one leg and not the other. If you do, one part of the body will be unbalanced and the whole idea of a massage is to give tone, balance and relaxation to the skin, muscles and nerves.

☐ Mold your hands to fit the area or contour of the body you are working on.

☐ When receiving a massage, let your mind become a blank. Let your entire body shift into neutral gear.

☐ Allow the person giving you the massage to move the various parts of your body. Do not try to help them as this will only cause you unnecessary muscle tension and defeat the purpose.

☐ Be aware of your body as it begins to feel liquid and rubbery.

☐ Let your body feel loose, like a soggy leaf on a wet log.

☐ Feel the tension, anxiety and worry slip away, fade, and disappear.

☐ If you feel like making sounds during the massage, do so.

☐ Get in tune with the sensation of simply floating and relaxing.

☐ Let's begin!

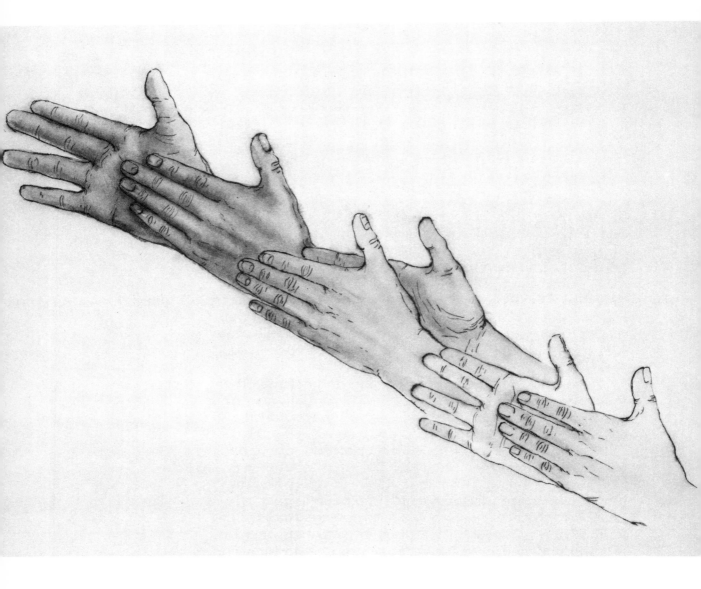

Warming Your Hands and Fingers Before a Massage

Never give a massage with cold or stiff hands. Warm them by palming, thumbing, and shaking, as described next.

palming

☐ Rub your palms together briskly until nice and warm. This is like rubbing your hands together on a cold day.

52

☐ Use the pad of your thumb to iron out the wrinkles **thumbing** on the palm and fingers of one hand. Then do this to the other hand.

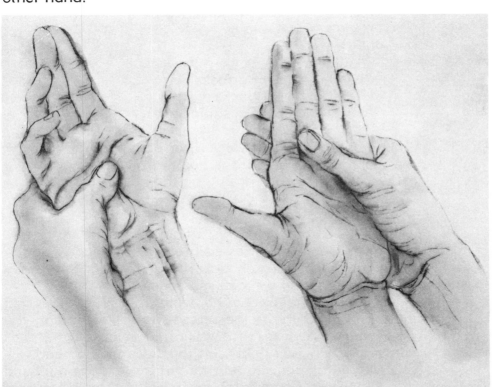

☐ Allow your arms to hang loosely at your sides. **shaking**
☐ Now vigorously shake both of your hands as if you are trying to shake sticky bubblegum or candy off the tips of your fingers.

To Begin You can start anywhere. However, this is the order I use most of the time:

Face	Stomach
Head	Legs
Neck	Feet
Shoulders	Back
Chest	Buttocks
Hands	Backs of Legs
Arms	Finishing Strokes

☐ Use only a few drops of oil for beginning on each of these areas. For parts of the body with lots of hair, use a little more oil to prevent pulling the hairs.

Facial Massage

The face is a good place to start since massaging it helps to unwind our tired, stressed brains. One nice variation when you don't have enough time to give a total body massage is to give a facial massage.

☐ First, soak one towel in hot water (not boiling). Wring it out and mold it onto the person's face leaving only the nose exposed. Leave the towel in place for 2–3 minutes holding your hands lightly on the sides of the head.

☐ Next, wring out a towel that has been soaking in cold (not ice) water. Remove the hot towel and mold the cold towel onto the face as before. Let the cold towel remain in place for 1 minute.

☐ Remove the cold towel and gently rub some oil, cream or lotion into the face.

☐ Then proceed with the face, head and neck massage movements on pages 55–75.

54

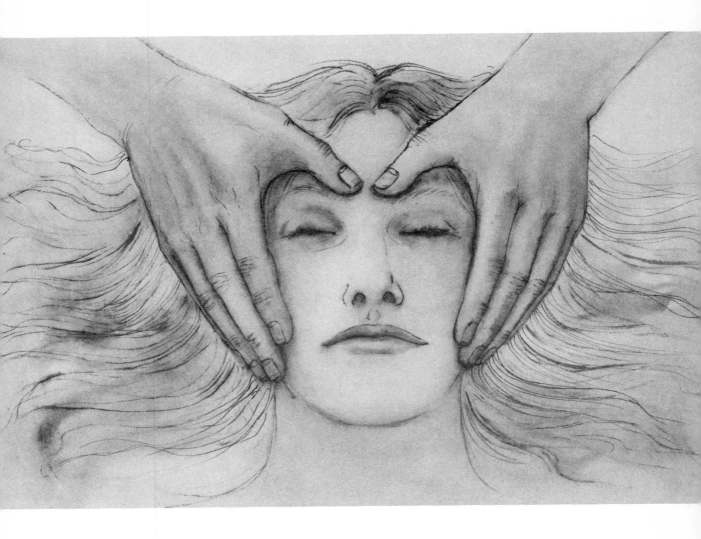

□ This movement is important since it is the first hand-to-body contact.

□ Make sure your hands are nice and warm. Gently place your open hands on the person's cheeks, allowing your thumbs to rest on the forehead.

□ This movement provides a nice energy exchange between the giver and receiver.

□ (1 minute) □

**laying on
of the hands**

□ The approximate time or number of strokes required for learning a particular movement is listed in parentheses. Once you have given several massages you may adjust the time or number of strokes to suit the needs of your partner. Never rush through a massage.

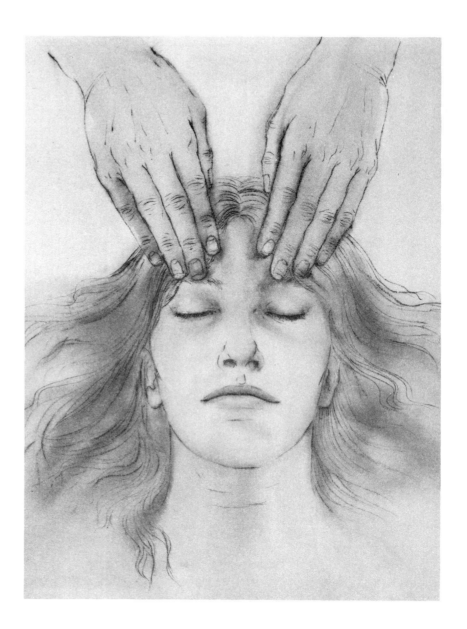

forehead oval ☐ Place the pads of the fingertips of both your hands on the person's forehead. Slowly make egg-shaped movements, starting from the middle of the forehead and progressing to the temples and sides of the head.
☐ Pressure should be light to medium.
☐ (3 times).

56

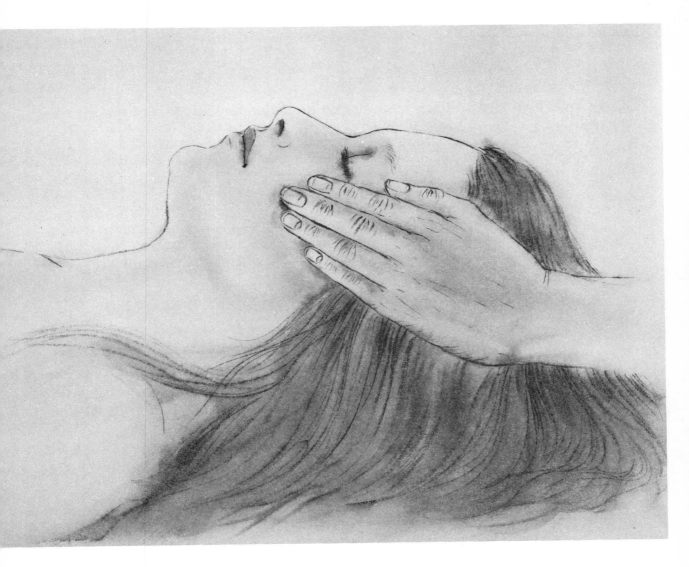

☐ Place your fingers on the person's cheeks and slowly **rosy cheeks** make circular motions on and around the cheeks.
☐ Feel the skin slide over the cheeks and jawbone.
☐ (3 times).

cheek boning ☐ Place your fingertips under the person's cheekbones and slowly but firmly pull the skin alongside both cheekbones toward the base of the ears.
☐ (3 times).

chin and jawbone pull ☐ Same as CHEEK BONING, except in this case place the ends of your fingers under the person's chin and jaw. Slowly pull the skin along the underside of the jawbone until you reach the ends of the jawbone near the ears.
☐ (3 times).

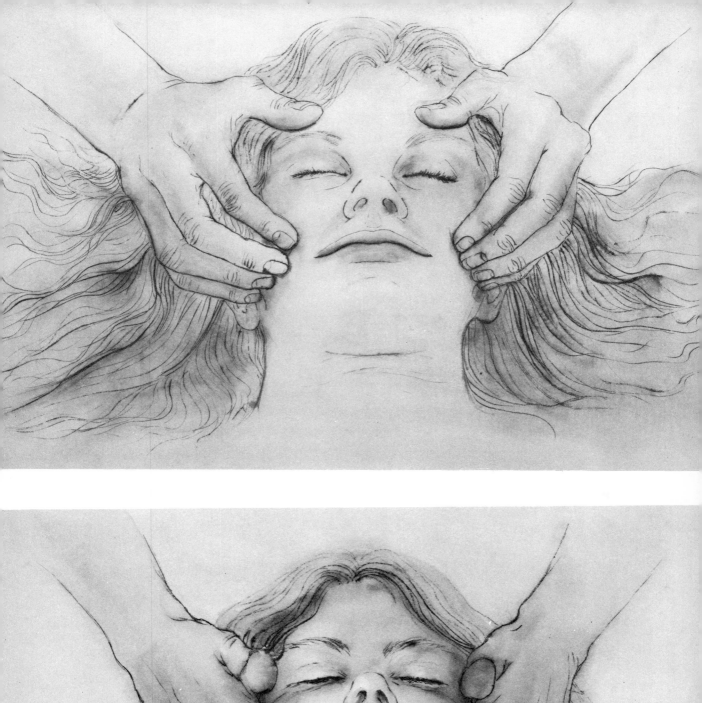
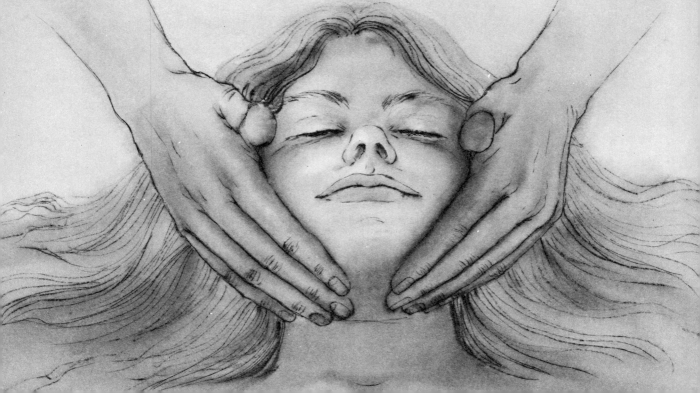

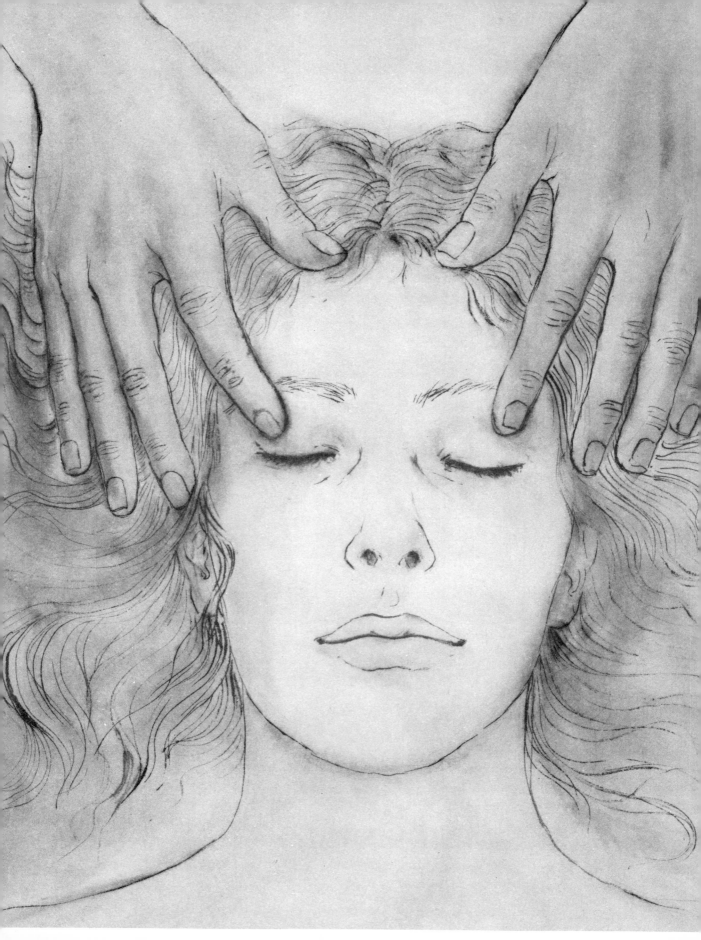

☐ Use the pads of your forefingers to ever-so-lightly **eyelid brush** brush the closed eyelids.
☐ (3 times).

Caution: Do not use oil on the eyelids.

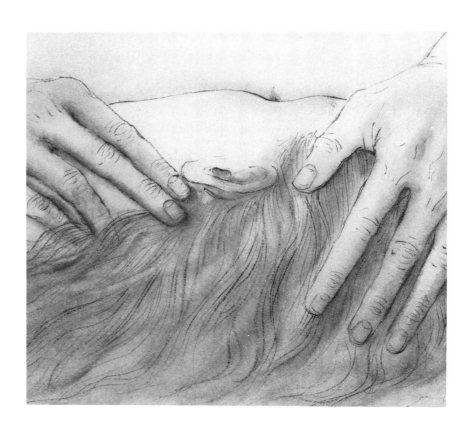

ear rings   ☐ Use the pads of your first two fingers to apply firm pressure while curving around the boney area behind the ear.
☐ (6 times).

☐ Go around the outside of the ear, using the same two fingers but applying lighter pressure.
☐ (6 times).

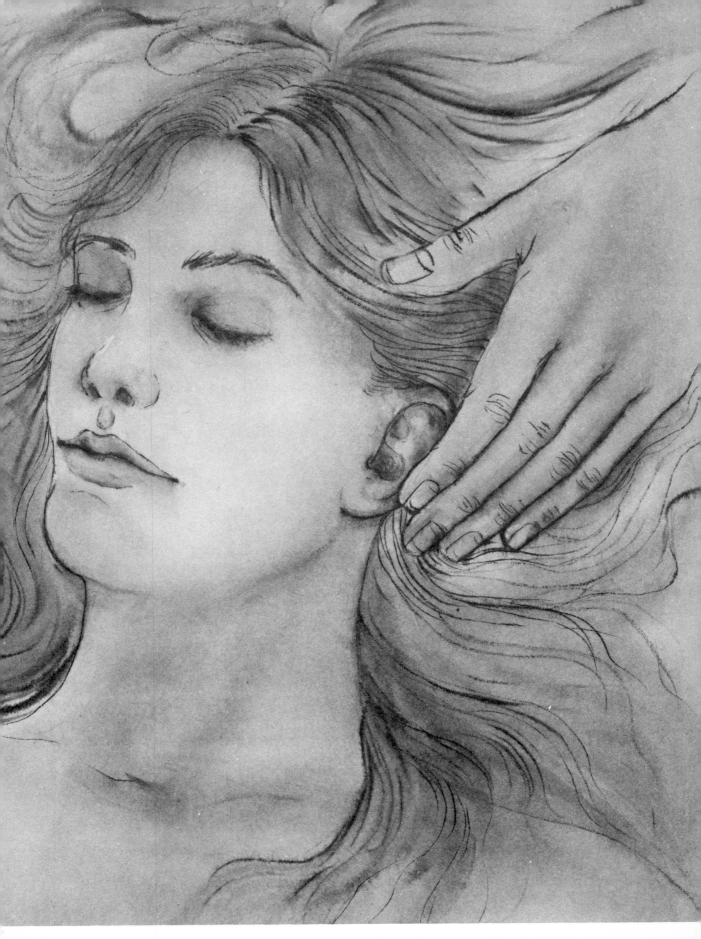

lip stick   □ Use the pad of one forefinger to make three complete circles around the edge of the person's lips. Now, make three gentle circles on the top surface of the lips.

□ Pressure should be very light. Like a butterfly landing on a leaf.

Head

head scratch   □ Use the tips of your thumbs and your fingertips to massage all over the tops and sides of the person's head. This is like giving someone a shampoo.

□ (1 minute).

Caution: When performing movements in which the head, arms or legs are elevated off the table or floor, make certain that you have a secure grip on the part of the body you are working on. Unless the person is confident that you will keep head, arms and legs from falling, he or she won't be able to relax completely.

□ Important: Avoid ALL of the head and neck movements if there is a possibility that the person being massaged has any head, neck or upper back problems.

64

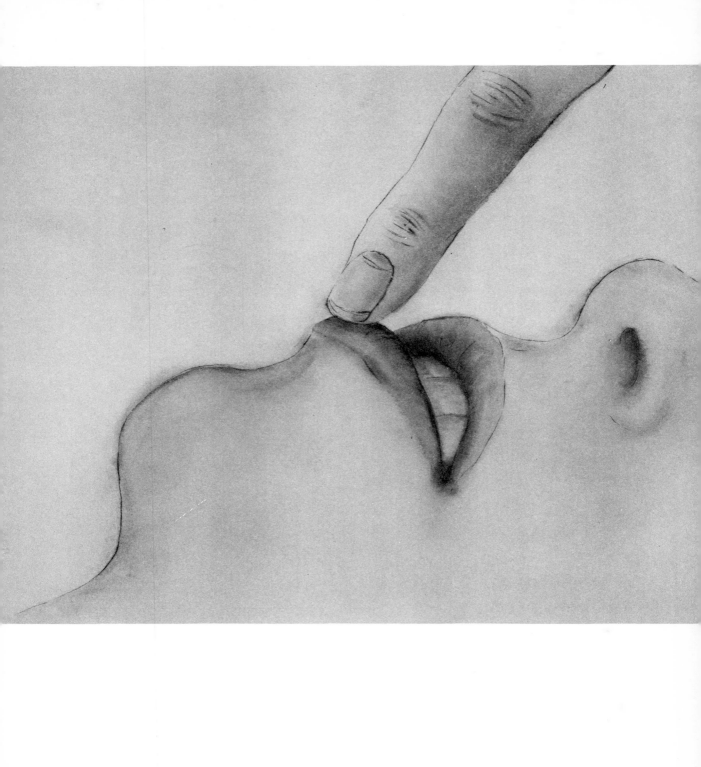

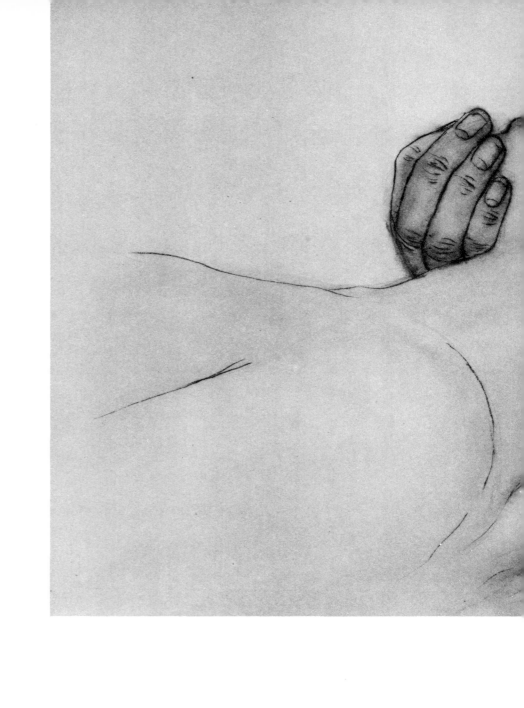

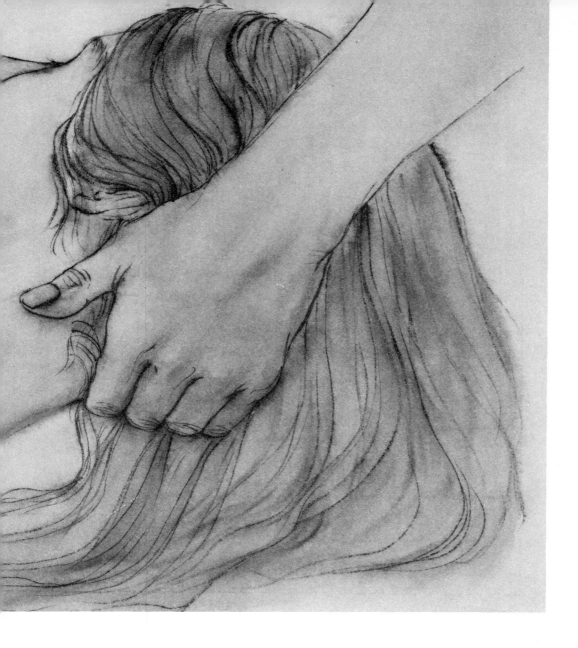

☐ Place one hand behind the head and the other hand **head rotation** under the chin. Elevate and support the head at a 45° angle to the person's body.

☐ Very, very slowly turn the head to the left side until a slight resistance is felt. Then slowly turn the head back to the center position. Now very slowly turn the head to the right and back.

☐ A very unusual and sensational movement.

☐ (3 complete rotations).

head sway   ☐ Slowly and gently move the head to one side until resistance is encountered or until the ear touches the top of the shoulder.
☐ Move the head to the other side.
☐ (2 complete sways).

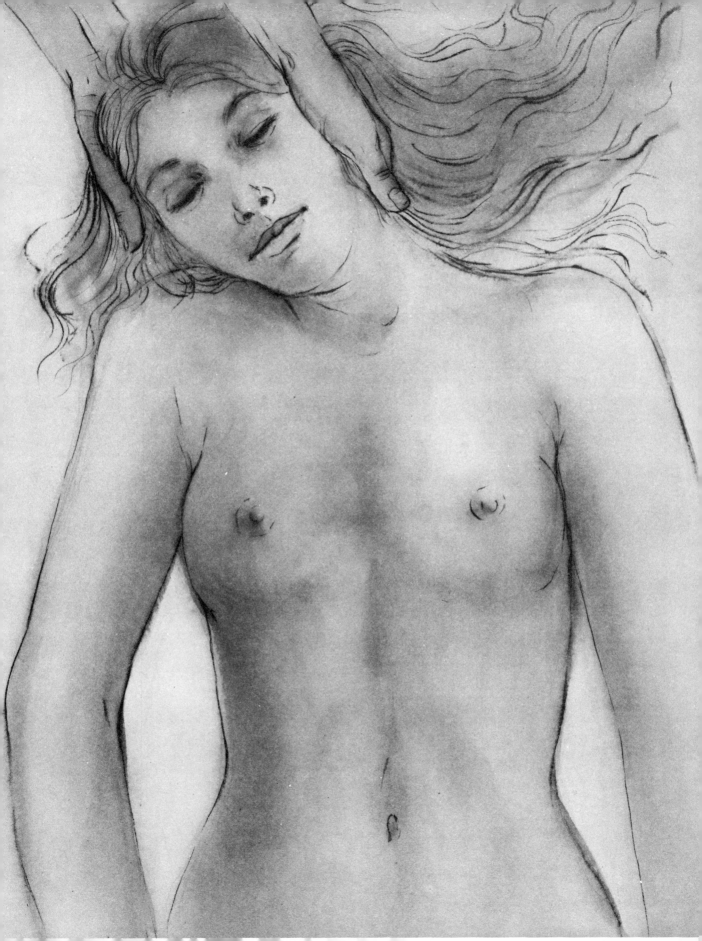

pushing a head ☐ Place your fingers back of the person's skull, with your thumbs alongside the head and slightly above the ears. Slowly and gently push the head forward until resistance is felt or until the chin touches the chest.

☐ Keep the head propped up in this position for a few seconds. GENTLY lower the head to its resting position and slowly withdraw your hands.

☐ (2 (times).

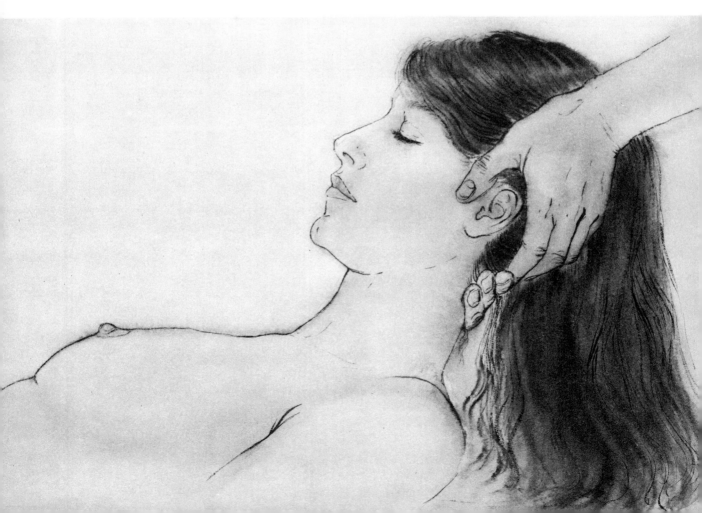

☐ Hold the person's head as you did in the illustration for HEAD ROTATION on page 66.

☐ Instead of rotating the head this time, GENTLY pull the head toward your body. Do not pull enough to move the whole body. Just pull until you feel some resistance. Then hold the head in this slightly stretched position for about 5 seconds.

☐ (3 times).

pulling a head

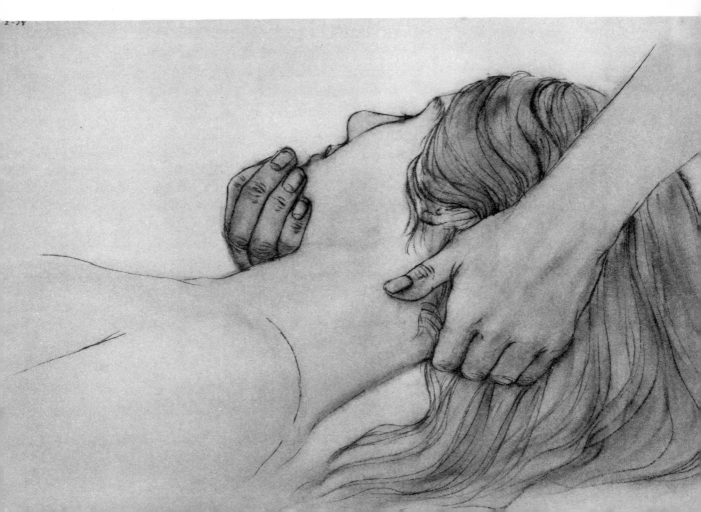

combing hair ☐ Spread your fingers into the shape of a comb. Beginning at the top of the forehead, run your fingers through the person's hair.
☐ Even though this feels good to most people, some may be finicky about having their hair messed up. In that case, omit this movement.
☐ (4 times).

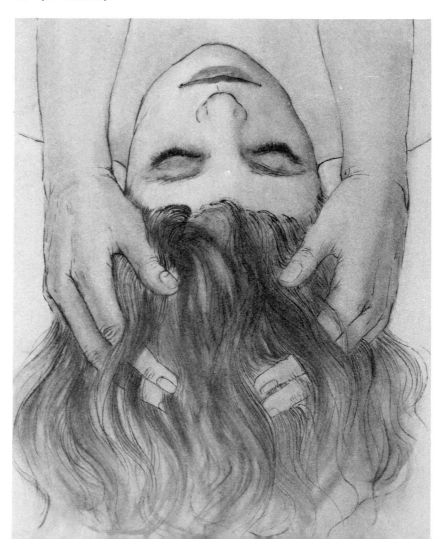

□ Use the fingers of each hand to make small circular movements starting from the shoulders and spiraling up along the back and sides of the neck to the base of the head.
□ (3 times).

neck spiral

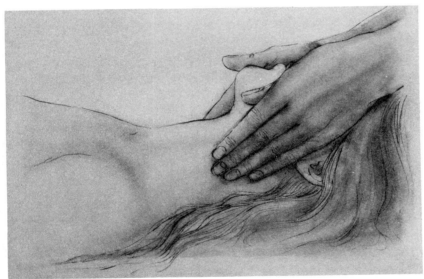

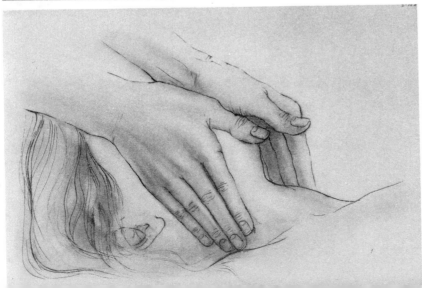

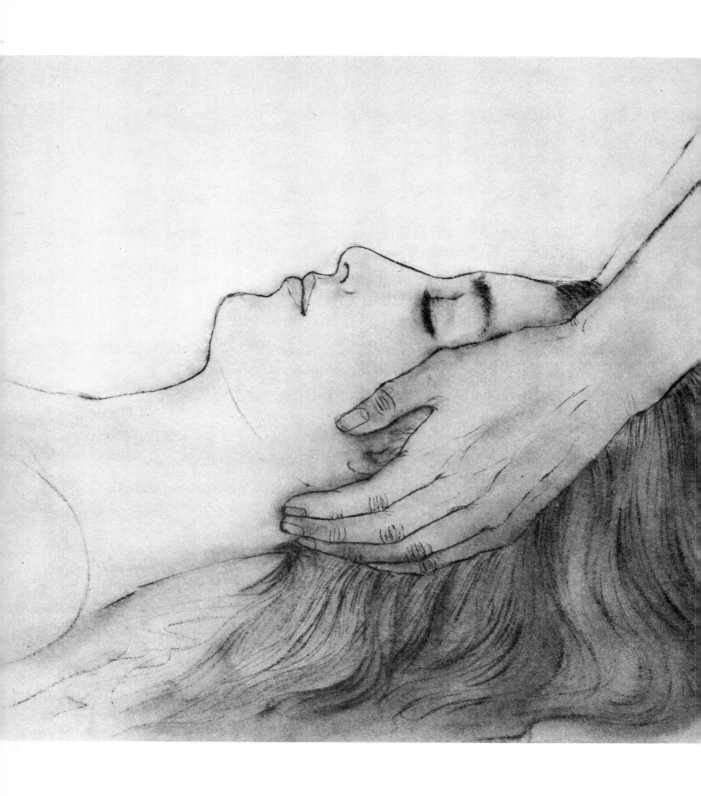

☐ Place the first two fingers of each hand into the two **neck vibration** indentations at or just below the base of the skull (where the back of the neck joins the skull).
☐ Make the ends of your fingers vibrate at a medium speed. Pressure should be firm but not painful.
☐ This movement helps to relieve tension.
☐ (30 seconds to 1 minute).
☐ Here is what this movement looks like when viewed from the back of the head.

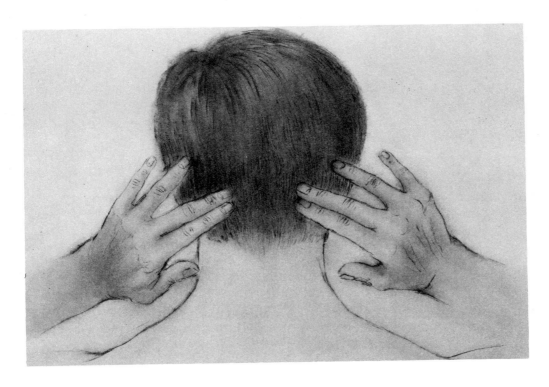

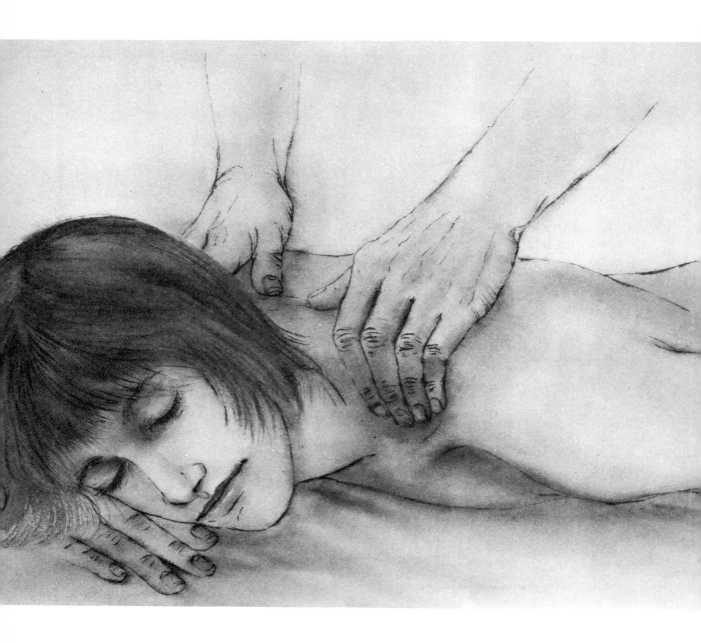

Shoulders

**taking a load
off the shoulders**

☐ Place your fingertips over the collar bones with the pads of your thumbs just above the shoulder blades.
☐ Slowly work your fingertips and thumbs into the muscle tissue by making gentle rocking and vibrating movements.
☐ (1–2 minutes).

76

☐ Place your fingertips on the underside of the person's **piano roll blues** shoulders. Lightly dig your fingertips into the shoulder muscles.

☐ Tap into the muscles all over the shoulder area. It's like playing the scale on a piano keyboard.

☐ (1–2 minutes).

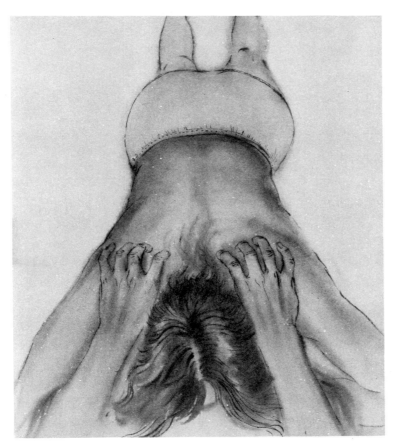

shoulder squeeze   □ Place your hands over the tops of the shoulders and squeeze several times.
□ Use medium pressure. It's like squeezing a softball.

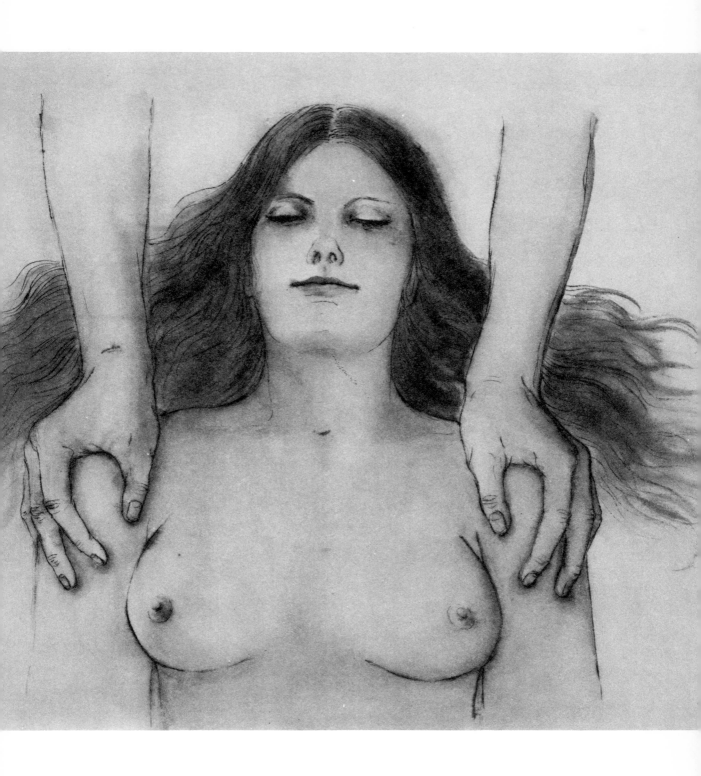

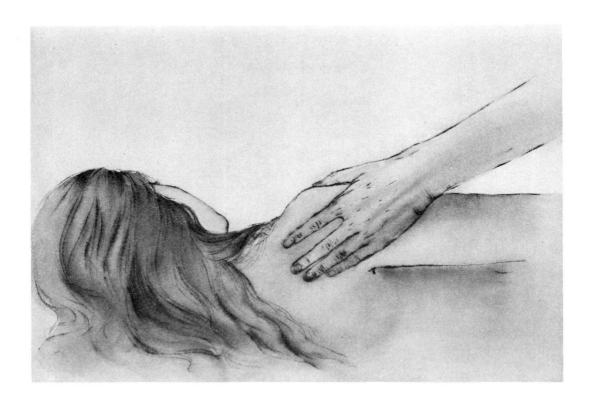

shoulder rotation   ☐ Lift up one shoulder and rotate clockwise (3 times) and counterclockwise (3 times).
☐ Now do the other shoulder.

Chest

midline slippery slide   ☐ Stand or kneel, depending on whether you are using a table or the floor, behind the person's head and place the palms of both your hands on the midline of the chest. Your hands should be side by side.
☐ Using medium pressure, slide down the chest and over the abdominal region to the pubic area.
☐ Mold your hands to fit the body contour and return by climbing along the rib cage and over the shoulders to the starting point.
☐ (3 times).

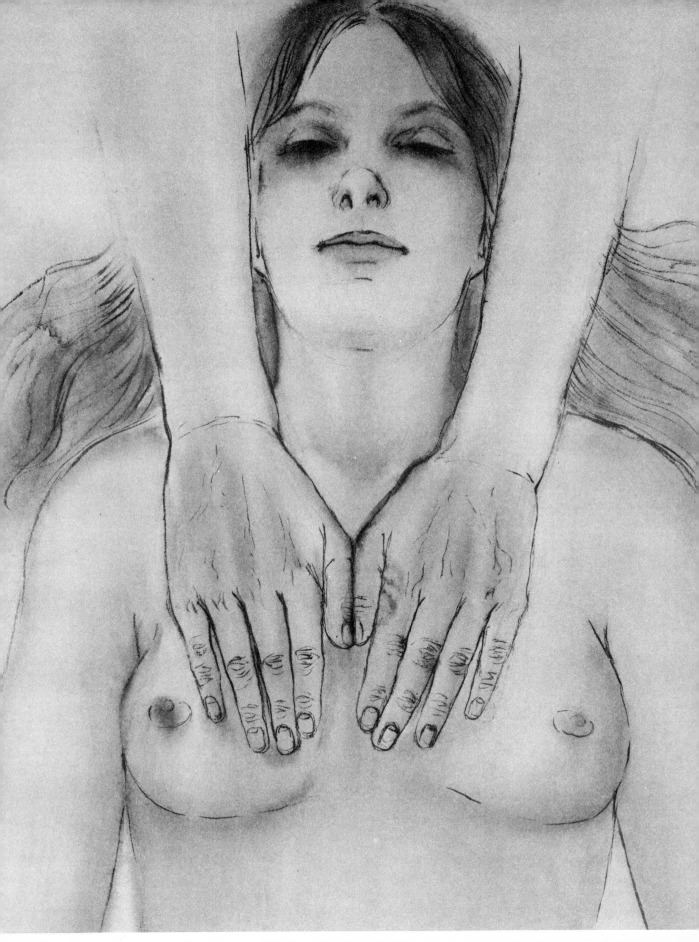

chest racetrack ☐ Place both of your hands flat on the outer part of the person's rib cage.

☐ Use light-medium friction to move in an oval race-track pattern going around the outside of the breasts, over the top of the chest and around the bottom of the abdominal region.

☐ (3 times).

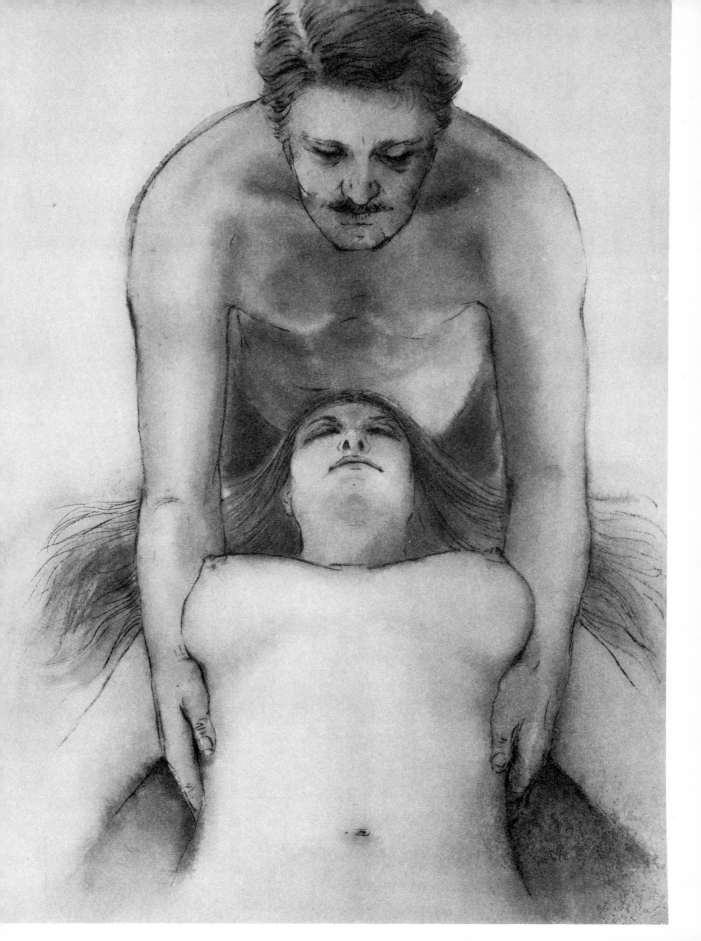

breast cupping ☐ Cup both of your hands over the breasts (male or female) and gently knead and squeeze several times.

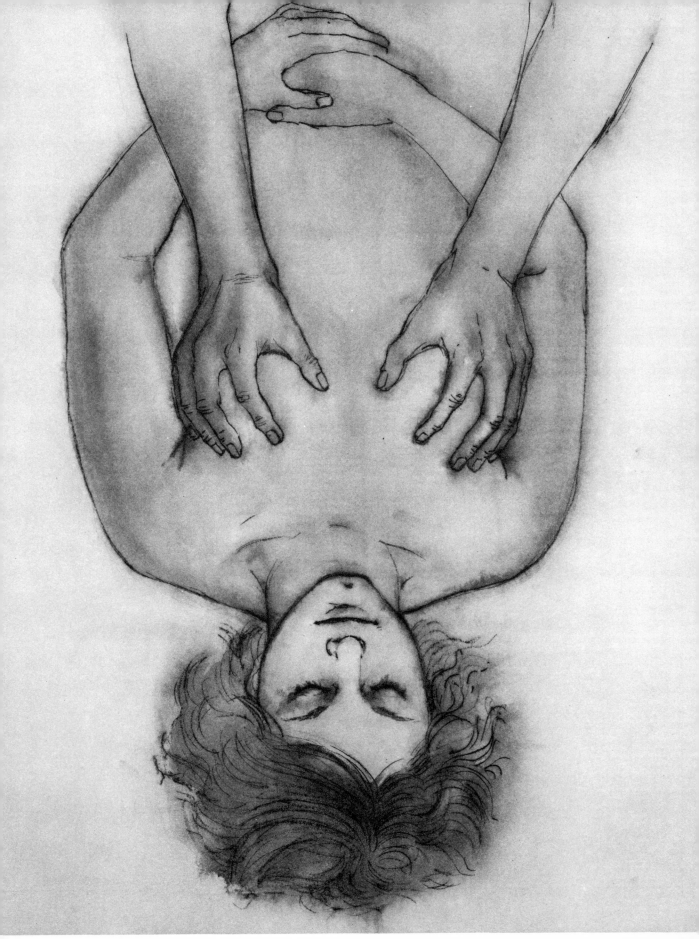

Hands

holding hands   ☐ Sandwich the person's hand between the palms of your own hands.
☐ (Hold still for 1 minute).
☐ Do one hand and then the other.

palm springs twist   ☐ Everybody's winner!
☐ With one hand cushion the person's hand from the back. With the heel of the other hand twist into and all around the palm of the person's hand.
☐ (1 minute).

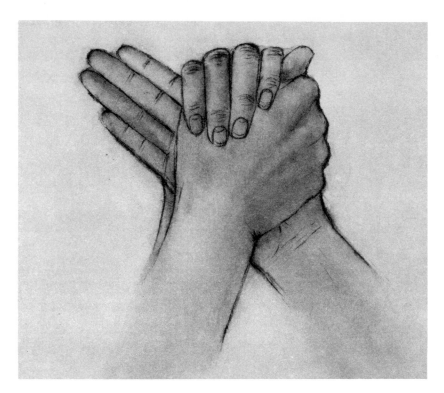

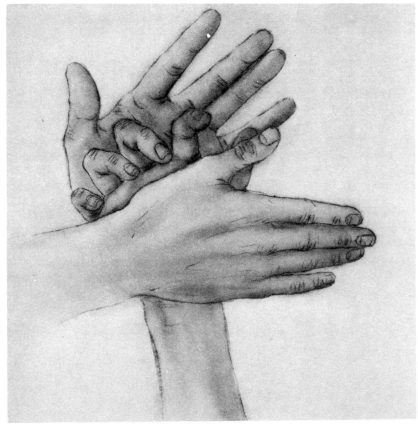

hand kneading   ☐ Place the pads of your thumbs on the back of the person's hand and place the pads of your fingers on his or her palm.
☐ Work your thumbs and fingers between the bones of the hands using flexible but firm pressure.
☐ (1–2 minutes).

ironing out hand   ☐ This movement was designed to "iron out" all those difficulties in the heel of the hand.
☐ Place the pads of your thumbs on the heel area of the hand.
☐ Use medium friction pressure to smooth out the wrinkles and difficulties in the heel of the hand.
☐ (1 minute).

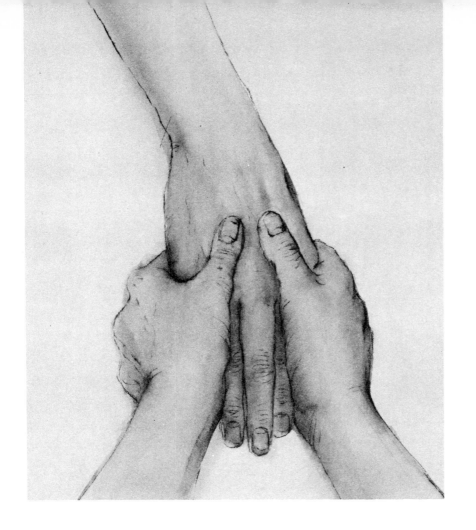

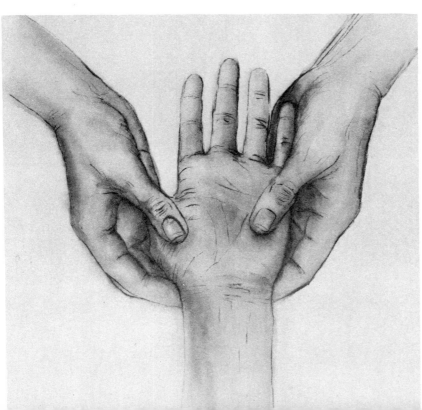

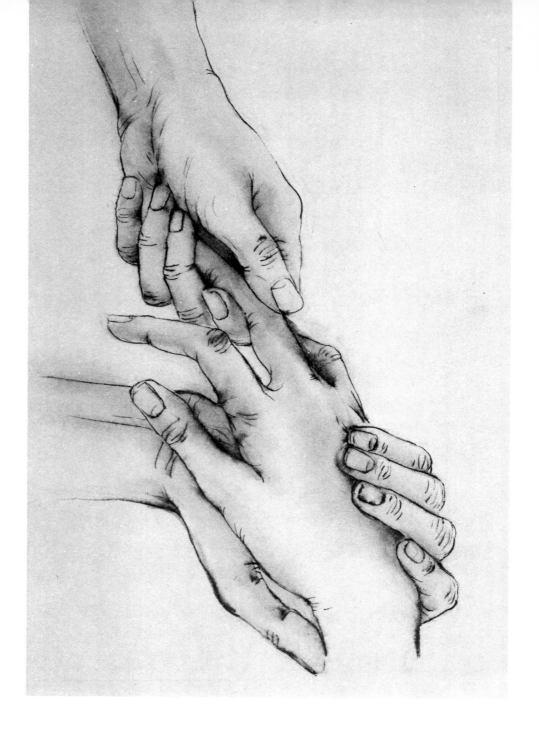

finger corkscrew ☐ Use your thumb and forefinger to corkscrew up and down each finger and thumb.
☐ Use firm pressure.
☐ (3 times for each finger and thumb).

90

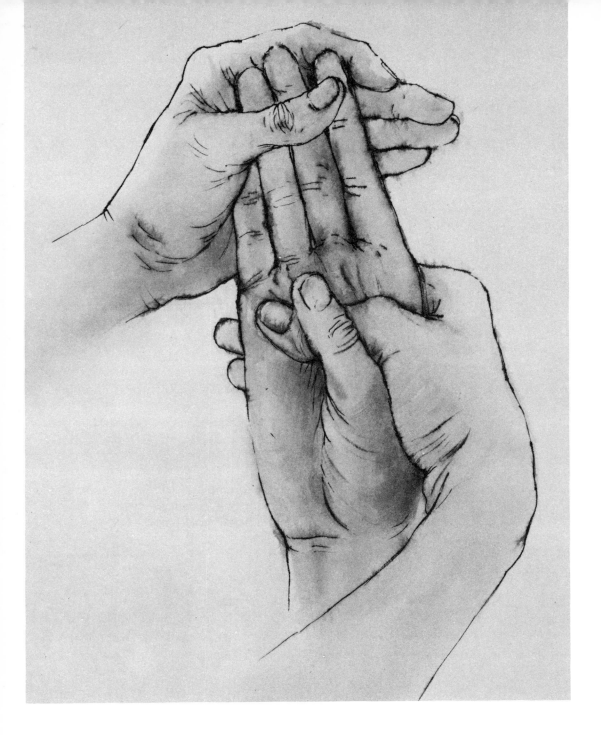

☐ Grasp the top part of the person's four fingers be- **finger rotation**
tween your thumb and fingers. Rotate clockwise and
counterclockwise.
☐ (3 times each way).

wrist rotation ☐ Same hold as in the FINGERS ROTATION, except make the whole hand rotate at the wrist instead of at the knuckles. Rotate clockwise and counterclockwise. ☐ (3 times each way).

hand back thrust ☐ Place your palm against the person's palm and slowly push back until resistance is felt. ☐ Hold at this point and gently rock back and forth. ☐ (10 seconds).

hand forward thrust ☐ Place your palm on the back surface of the person's hand. Push forward until resistance is felt. ☐ Hold at this point and rock back and forth. ☐ (10 seconds).

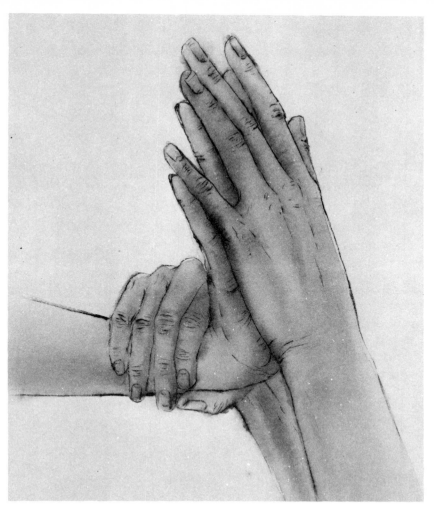

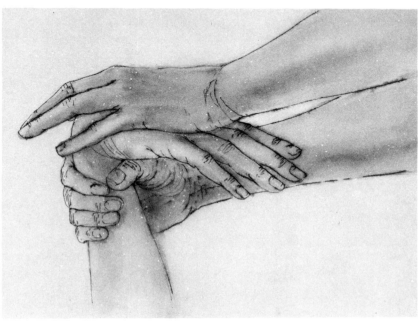

hand toothpaste squeeze

☐ A different stroke folks will like.
☐ Grasp the person's hand with your thumbs on the top of his or her hand, just below the wrist. Place your fingers against the palm of his or her hand.
☐ Use a firm, squeezing pressure to slowly glide your hands all the way out to the ends of the fingertips. It is as if you are trying to squeeze toothpaste out of the hand.
☐ (3 times).
☐ Now, on the other hand . . .

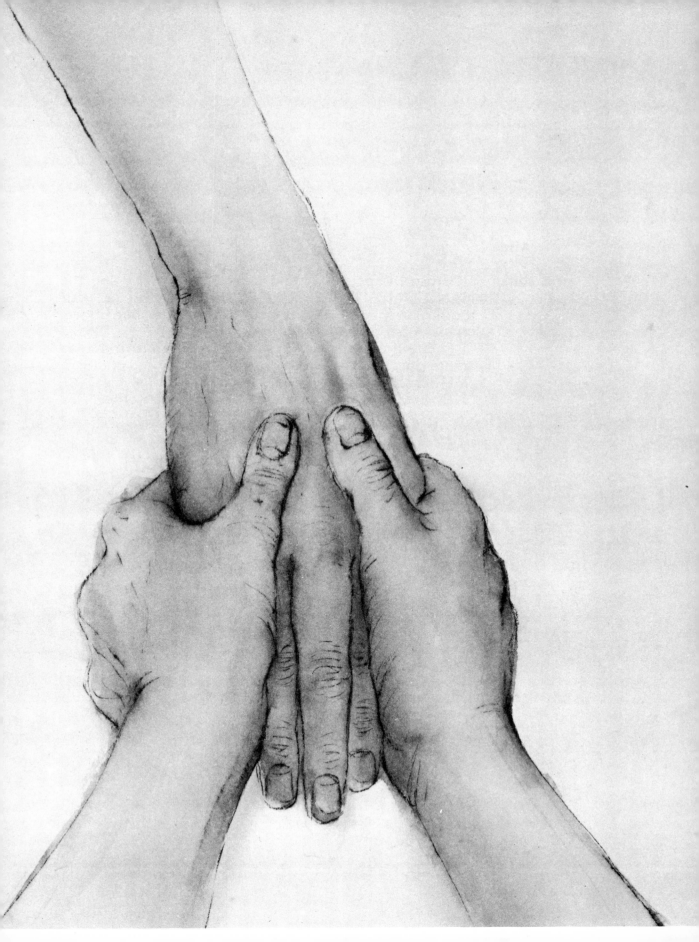

Arms

arm shake ☐ Grasp the person's hand as you did when doing the HAND KNEADING movement, page 88. Place your thumbs on the top of the person's hand and your fingers on his or her palm.
☐ Shake the arm up and down as if you are trying to create ripples in water or to rattle the links in a chain.
☐ (15 seconds).
☐ Do one arm entirely before working on the other.

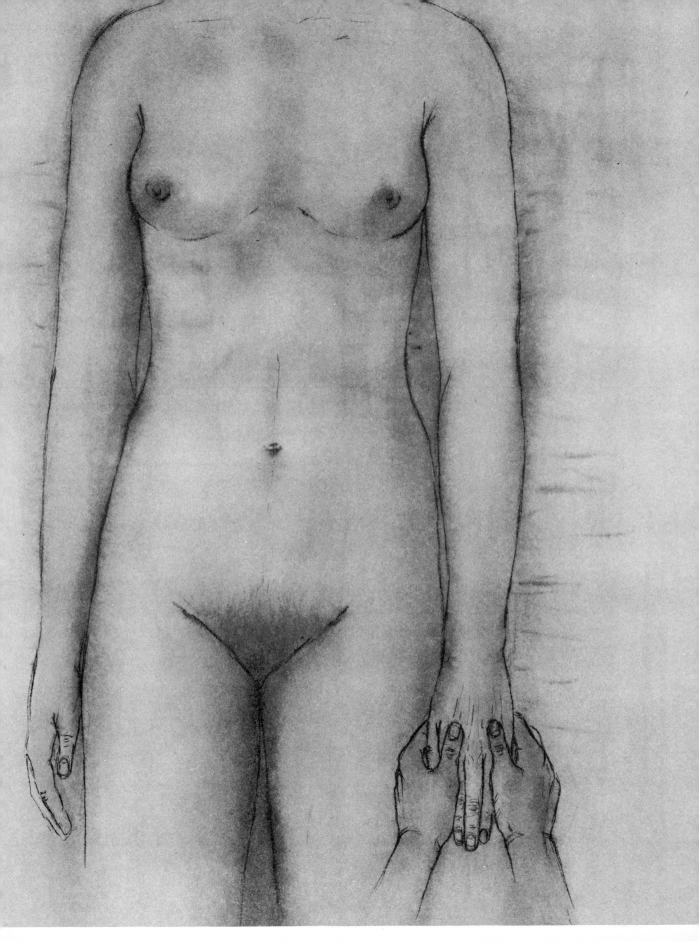

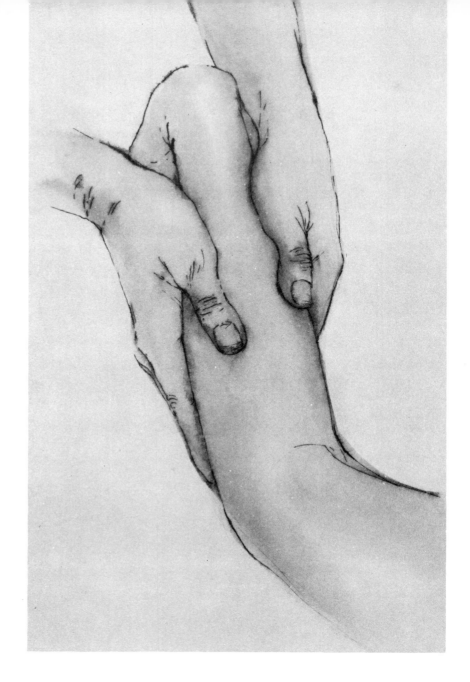

lower arm kneading ☐ With the person's elbow resting on the table or the floor, elevate the lower arm at about a 45° angle from the elbow.
☐ Place both of your hands around the wrist area. Use medium pressure and knead up and back from the wrist to the elbow.
☐ (3 times).

98

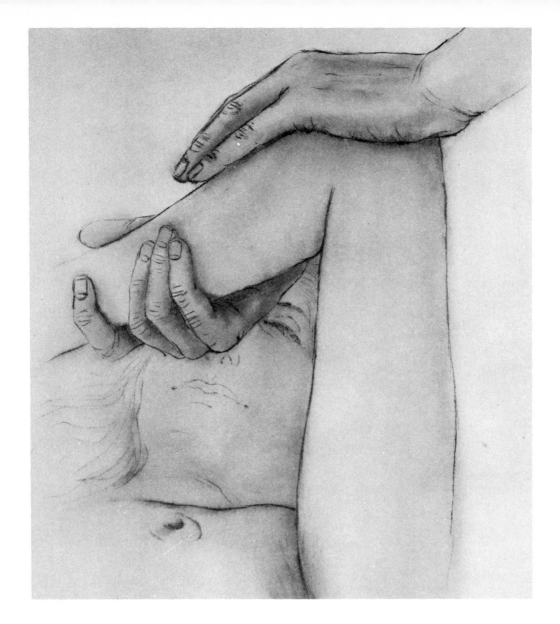

☐ Place the center of your palm against the person's elbow. Make small circles while pushing and twisting with your palm.
☐ (15 seconds).

elbow grease

☐ Place the person's hand between your rib cage and your upper arm and hold it in place. While holding the arm in place, knead the upper arm from elbow to shoulder. Use medium pressure.
☐ (3 times).

upper arm kneading

arm toss ☐ Grasp the person's arm and hold it straight up in a vertical position.
☐ Now toss the arm from one of your hands to the other hand. Be sure to catch the arm each time—do not let it drop.
☐ (12 times).

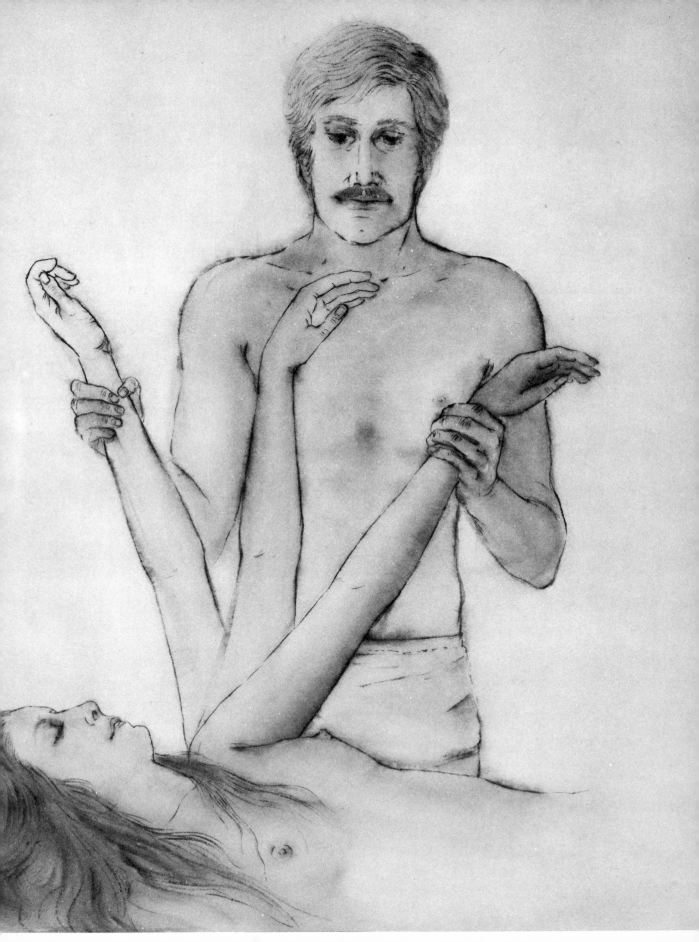

outside arm stroke	☐ Hold the person's wrist between your thumb and fingers. Lift the arm to a 45° angle.

☐ Mold your other hand to fit the arm and, using some friction, stroke from the wrist to the shoulder.

☐ Use a little more oil if the person has a lot of hair on his or her arm.

☐ (4 times).

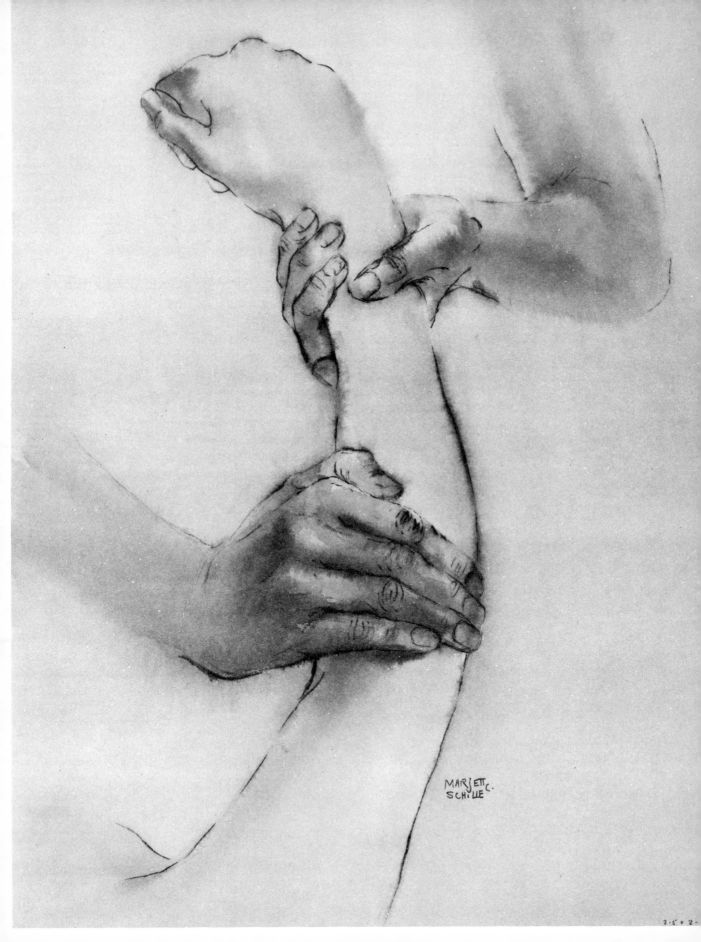

inside arm stroke   ☐ Same hold as the OUTSIDE ARM STROKE. Stroke the inside of the arm.
☐ (4 times).

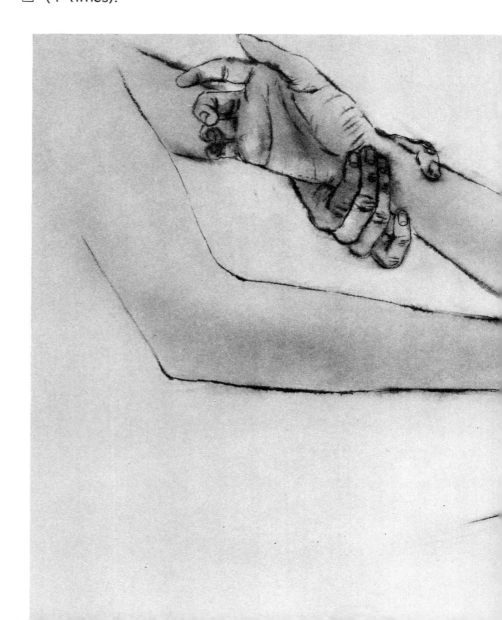

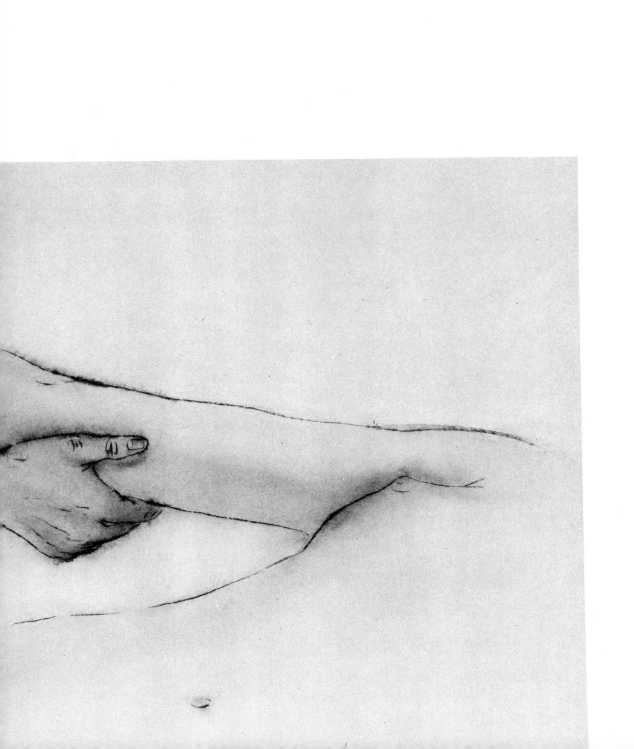

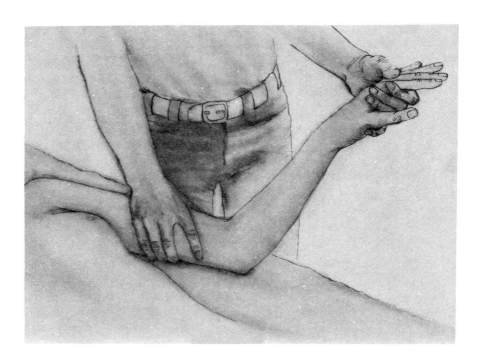

elbow rotation ☐ Hold the person's arm just above the elbow and rotate the lower arm in wide circles.
☐ Rotate clockwise and counterclockwise.
☐ (2 times each way).

arm stretching ☐ Grasp both arms at the wrists. Stretch both arms above the head.
☐ Pull on both arms until you can gently rock the person's entire body back and forth.
☐ Stimulates muscles and skin on the back of the body.
☐ (30 seconds).

106

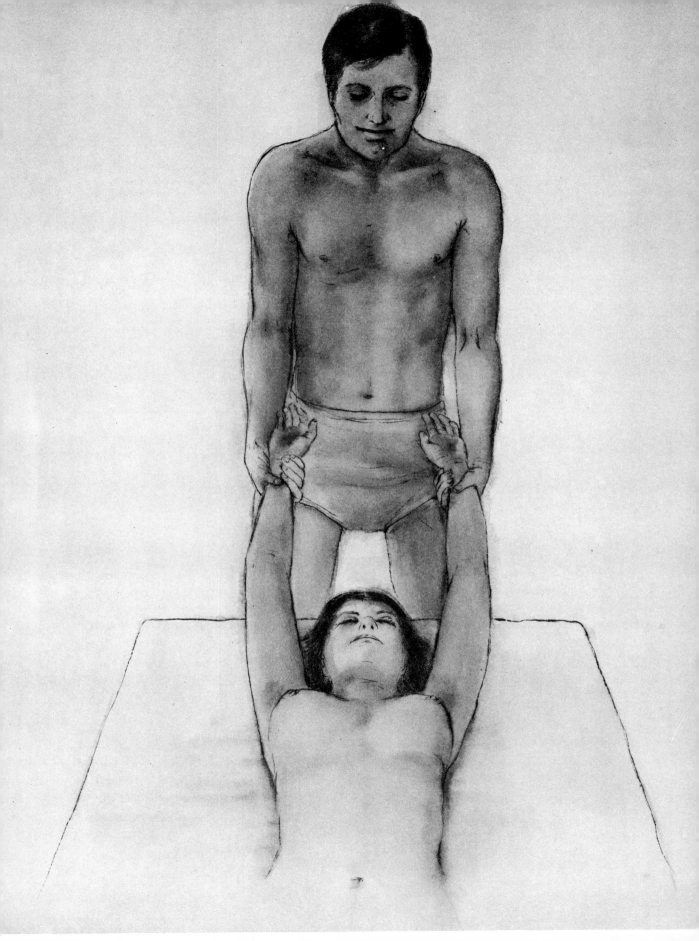

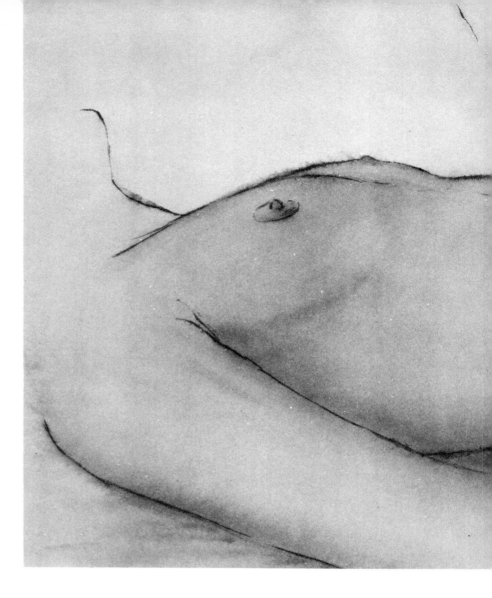

Stomach

stomach kneading   ☐ Flex the person's legs by placing the soles of the feet flat on the table or floor. This position serves to relax the muscles of the abdominal region.
☐ Gently dig your thumbs and fingers into the skin and muscle tissue. It's like kneading flour dough or pottery clay.
☐ (1 minute only).

Caution: Too much time spent on the abdominal region may result in the need for bowel elimination. This could be embarrassing during the massage but it's great for constipation.

108

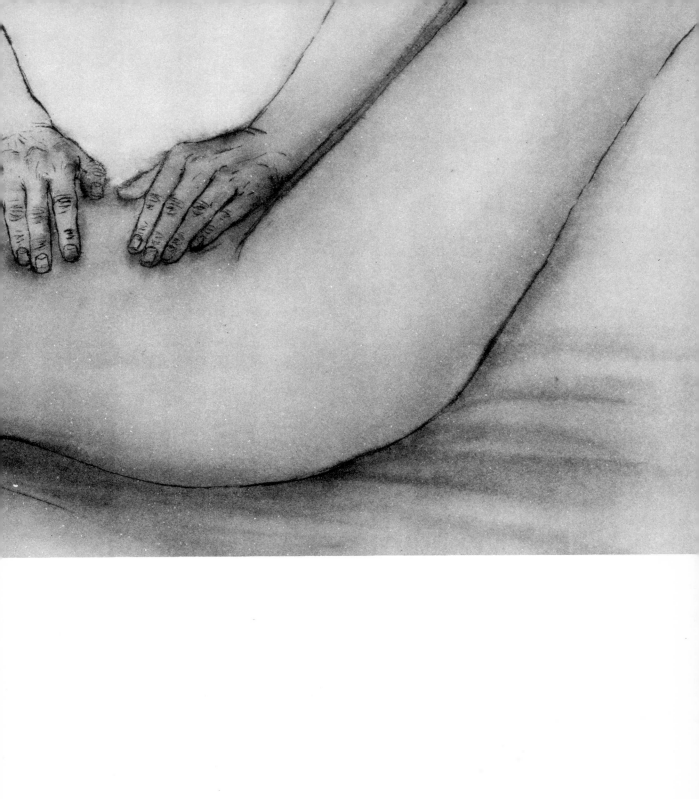

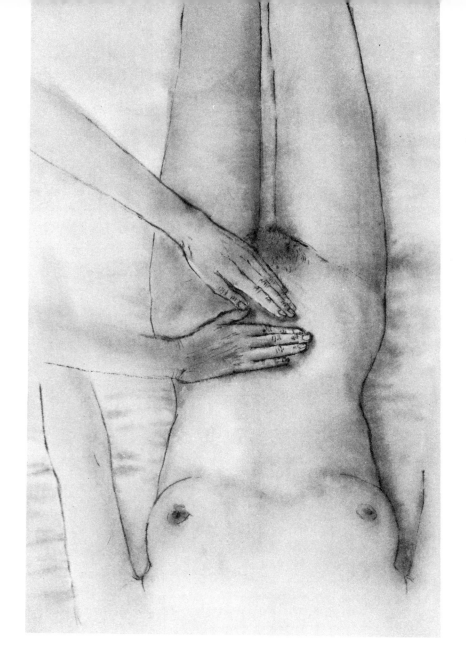

stomach rock ☐ Place the heels of your hands on the person's abdominal region. Keep your hands side by side.
☐ Alternately rock the heels of your hands gently back and forth all over the abdominal area. As you release the pressure with the heels of your hands, you can gently pull the skin toward you by using the pads of your fingers.
☐ Use medium pressure.
☐ (1 minute only).

110

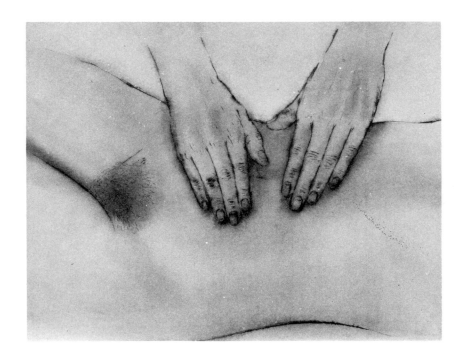

☐ Place the pads of the fingers of both your hands close **colon chase** together at the lower right-hand side of the person's abdominal region.

☐ Making little circles, follow the colon around the area below the rib cage and down to the pubic bone and back to the starting point.

☐ Use medium pressure. Go only in a CLOCKWISE direction.

☐ (3 times only).

111

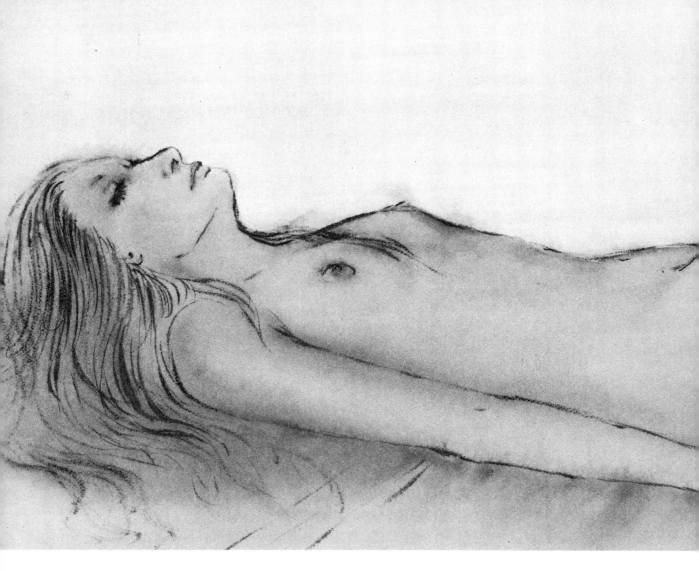

Legs

calf kneading

☐ Flex the person's legs by placing the soles of the feet on the table or floor.

☐ Grasp one leg about 6 inches above the ankle, using both of your hands. Work back and forth between the knee and the ankle.

☐ Use medium pressure.

☐ (4 times).

☐ Do one leg entirely before working on the other.

Caution: Do not knead directly under the knee.

112

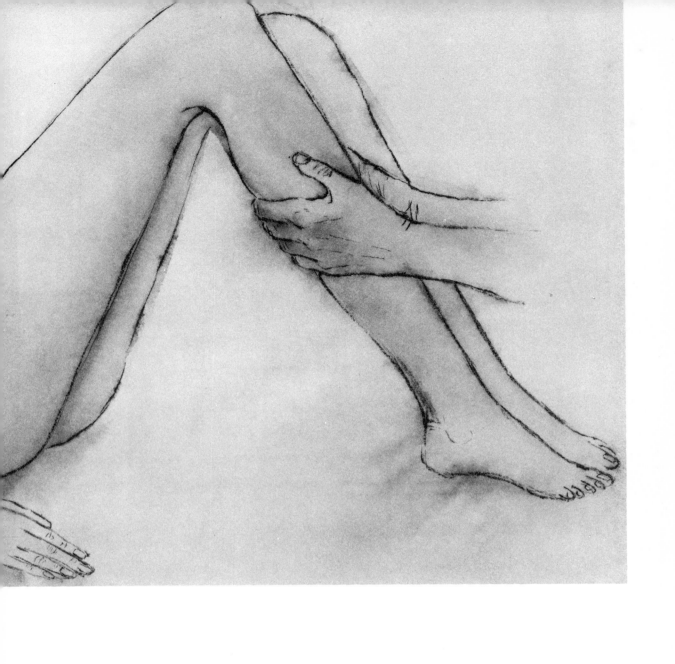

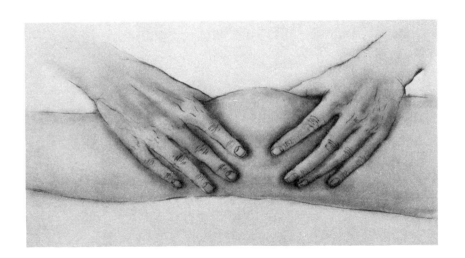

knee kneading ☐ Mold both of your hands around the outside of the person's kneecap. Stimulate the kneecap by causing your grip to pulsate once per second.
☐ (15 seconds).

kneecap rub ☐ Similar to the ELBOW GREASE, page 99.
☐ Place the palm of your hand on the person's kneecap and make circular movements while pushing in on the kneecap.
☐ Use medium pressure.
☐ (30 seconds).

114

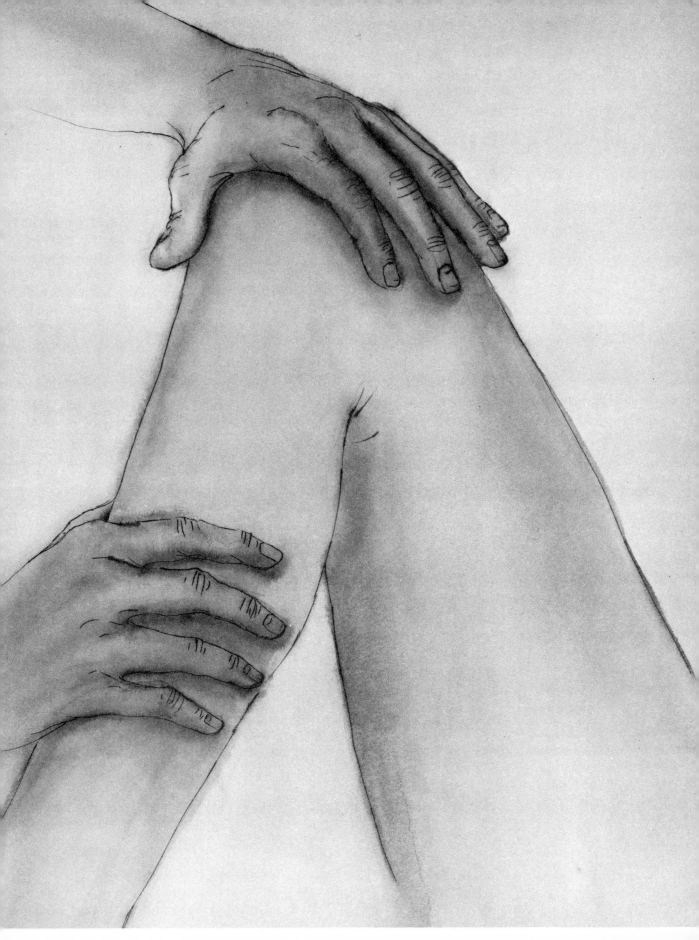

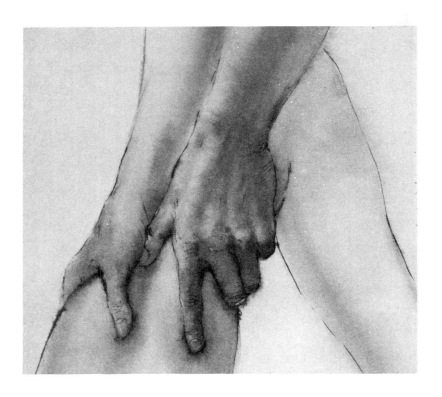

front thigh kneading ☐ Mold your hands around the lower thigh and work up an inch at a time until you reach the hip. Then work back down the thigh.
☐ Each time you return to the knee, move the position of your hands slightly and work up and back again.
☐ Use medium-heavy pressure.
☐ (4 times).

Variation: You can try rolling the skin of the thigh between your hands as you work your way up from the knee to the hip.

outside leg stroking ☐ Hold the person's leg just above the ankle. Lift the leg to a 45° angle.
☐ Mold your hand to fit the leg and, using some friction, stroke from the ankle to the hip.
☐ Use a little more oil if the person has a lot of hair on his or her legs.
☐ (4 times).

116

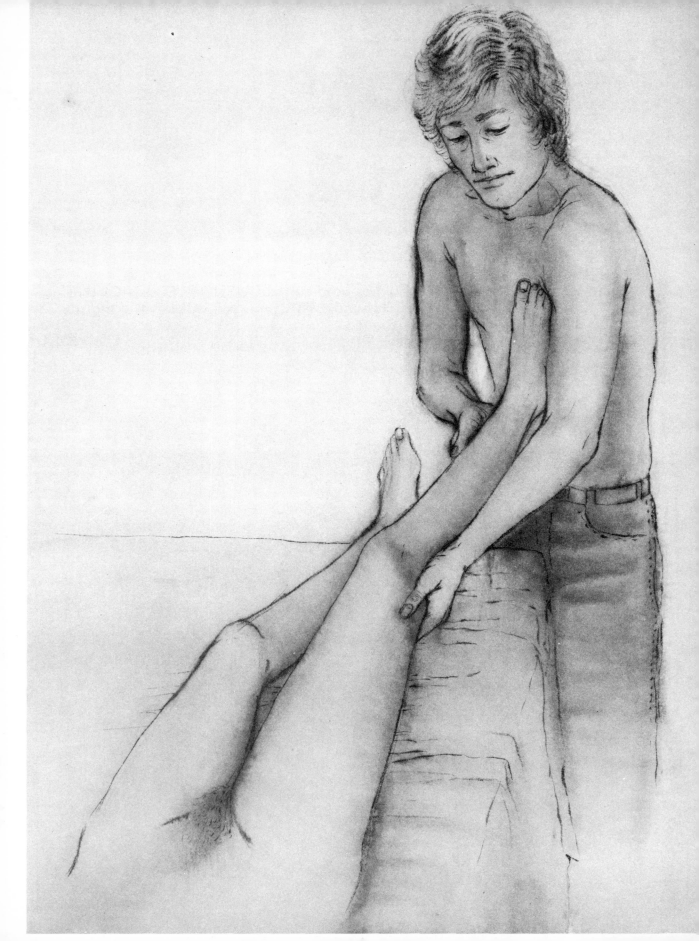

inside leg stroking   ☐ Same hold as used on the OUTSIDE LEG STROKING, except switch hands. This time you will be stroking the INSIDE of the leg.
☐ (4 times).

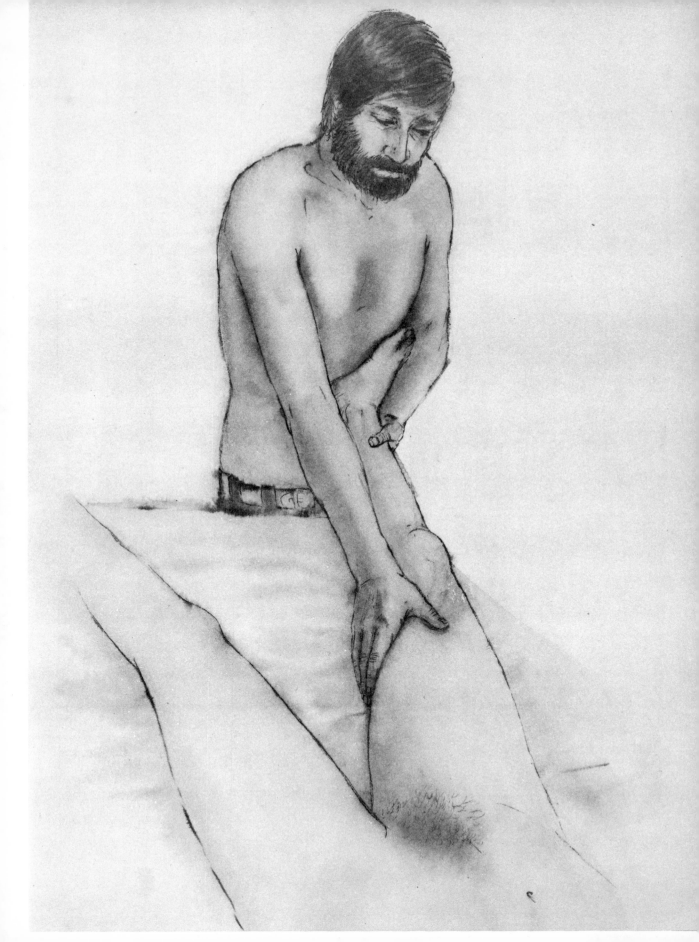

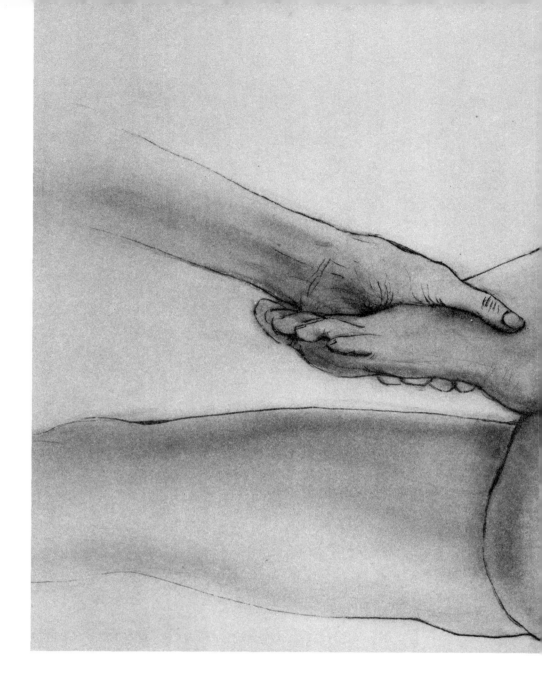

leg flexion   ☐ Grasp the person's foot with one hand and place your other hand on the person's knee. Push the leg back toward the body until resistance is felt.
☐ Hold the leg at this point and gently pump the leg toward the body for 15 seconds. Do not force the leg.
☐ When finished with the flexion movement, return the leg to its normal resting position.

120

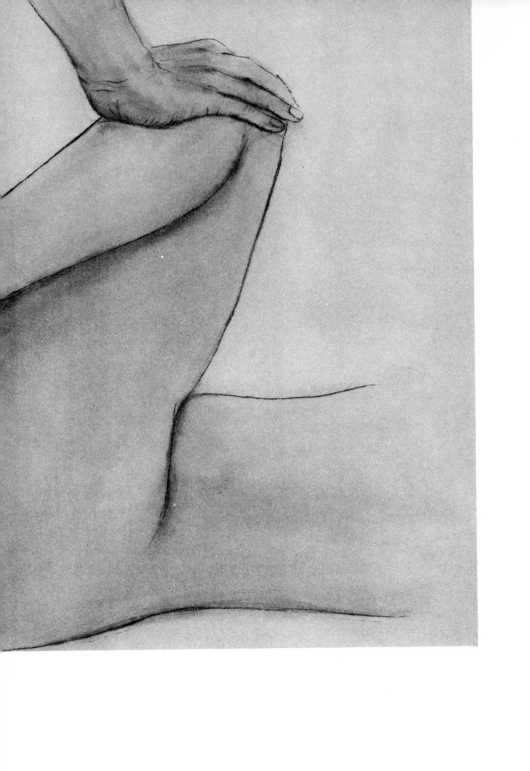

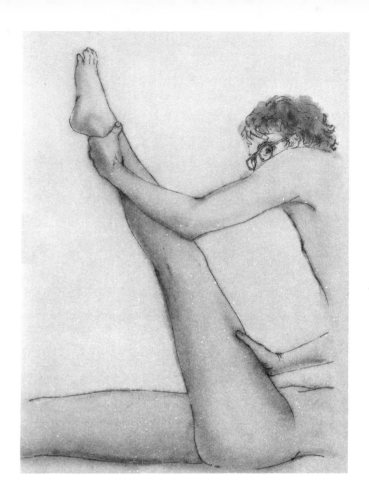

having a leg up ☐ Grasp the person's leg with one hand at the ankle and the other at the thigh.
☐ Extend the leg up and attempt to make a 90° angle to the body. Move the leg up toward the body until resistance is felt or until you notice that the knee of the other leg is rising off the table or floor. Do not force the leg.
☐ Hold the leg in that position for a few seconds.
☐ After you have finished, gently return the leg to its resting position, making certain not to drop it.

leg push-pull ☐ Grasp both legs just above the ankles with your hands on the backs of the person's legs.
☐ Alternately push and pull so that the entire body gently moves back and forth over the table or floor.
☐ This movement was designed to stimulate nerve endings in the back and buttocks.
☐ (15 seconds).

122

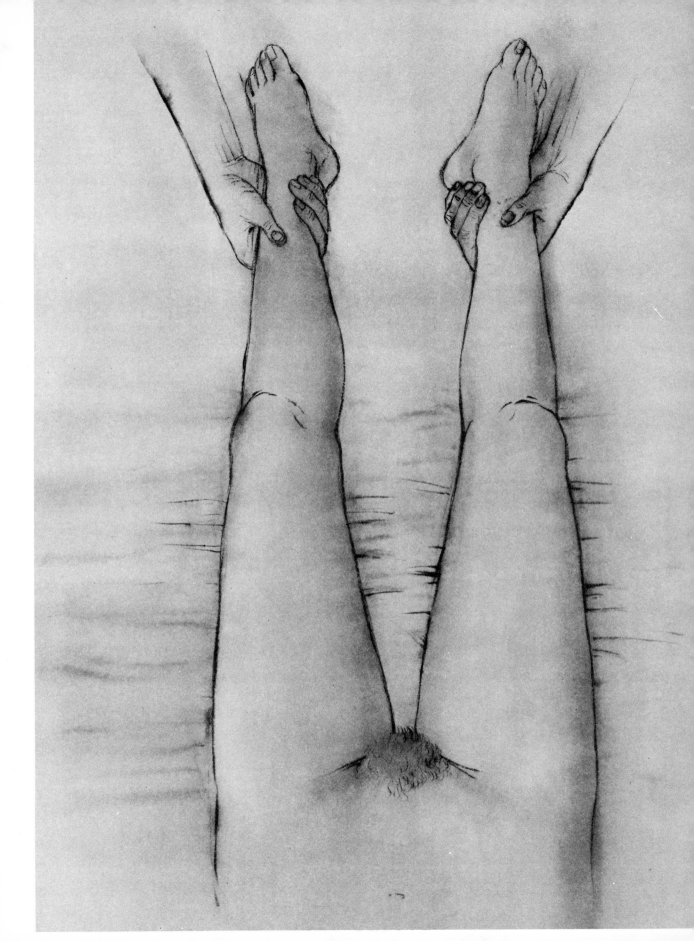

you're pulling my leg ☐ Same hold as used in the LEG PUSH-PULL movement.
☐ Do a low steady pull toward you and hold the person's legs at that point for 5 seconds.
☐ (3 times).

windshield wiper ☐ Grasp the person's legs as in the LEG PUSH-PULL movement. Turn the feet toward each other. (10 times). Turn the feet away from each other. (10 times).
☐ Turn both feet toward the right. (10 times). Turn both feet toward the left. (10 times).
☐ When finished with these movements, return the legs to their resting position.

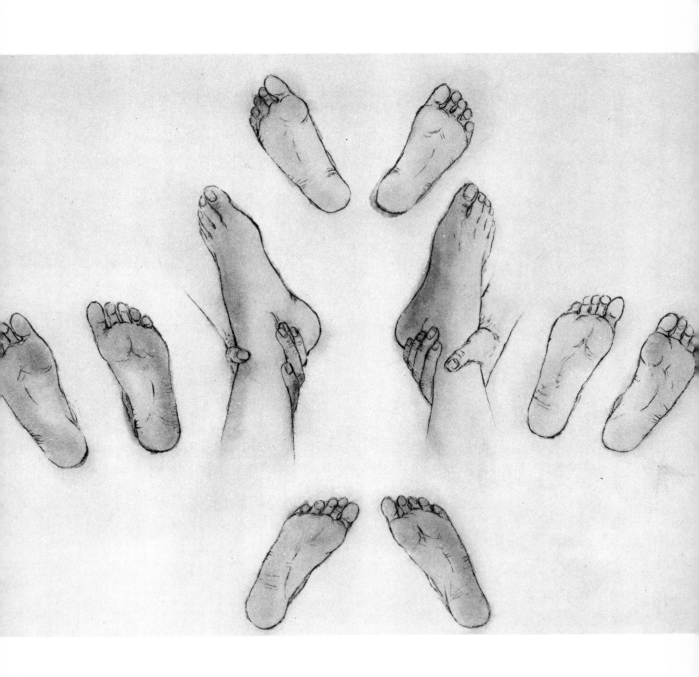

Feet

getting a foot hold ☐ Simply sandwich the person's foot between the palms of your hands and hold it there quietly for 30 seconds.
☐ Do one foot and then the other.

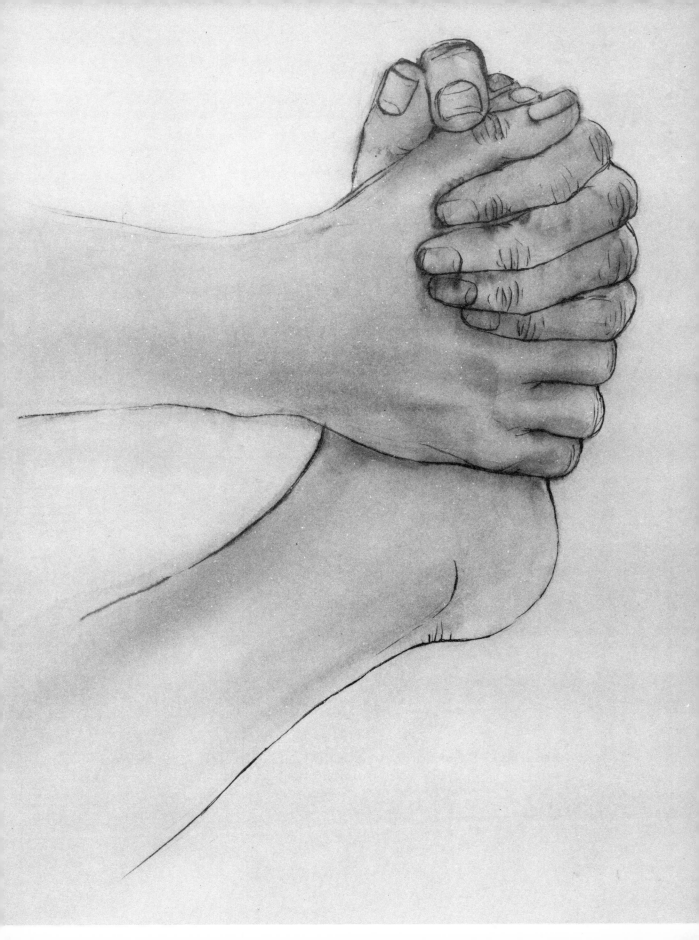

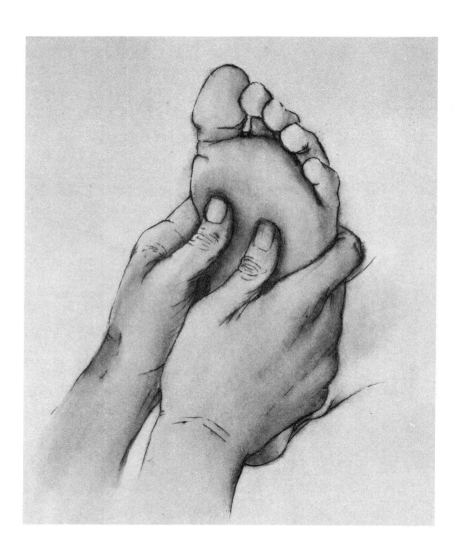

foot kneading ☐ Similar to the HAND KNEADING movement, page 88.
☐ Work your thumbs and fingertips between the small bones of the person's foot.
☐ (1 minute).

128

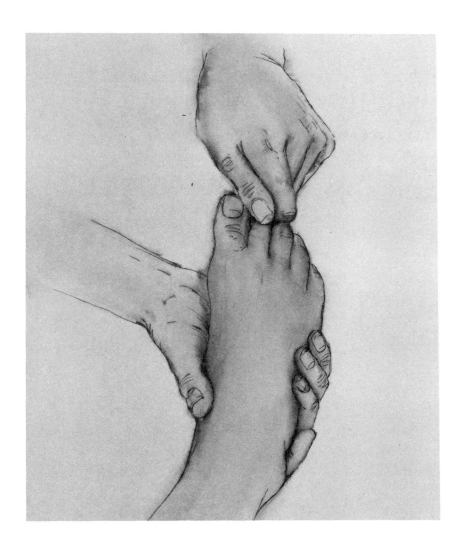

☐ Use your thumb and forefinger to corkscrew up and **toe corkscrewing**
down each toe.
☐ Use firm pressure.
☐ (3 times on each toe).

129

toe rotation ☐ Grasp the top part of the toes of one foot using your thumb and fingers. Rotate clockwise and counterclockwise.
☐ (3 times each way).

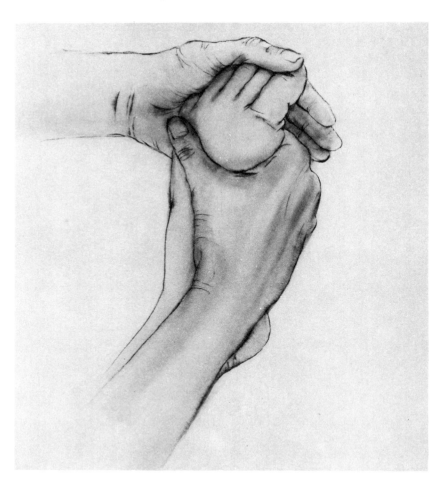

☐ Grasp the toes with one hand and the ankle with your other. Make the whole foot rotate at the ankle. Rotate clockwise and counterclockwise.
☐ (3 times each way).

ankle rotation

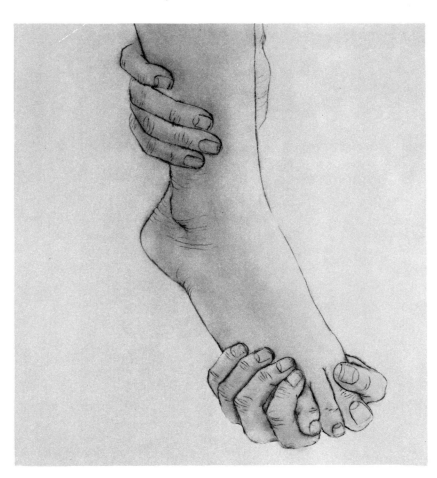

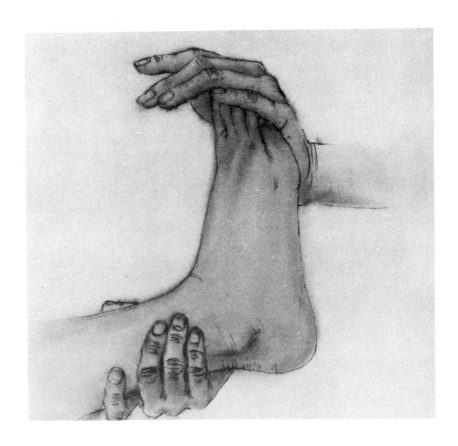

foot back thrust ☐ Place your hand flat over the sole of the person's foot. Slowly push back until some resistance is felt.
☐ Hold the foot at this point and gently rock it back and forth several times.

132

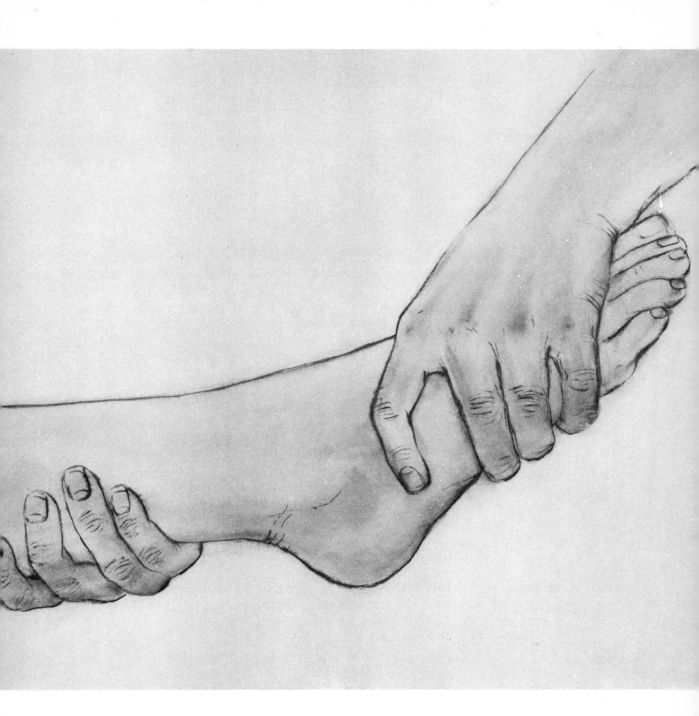

□ Grasp around the top of the person's foot near the **foot forward thrust**
toes. Push forward until some resistance is felt.
□ Hold the foot at this point and gently rock it back
and forth for a few seconds.

133

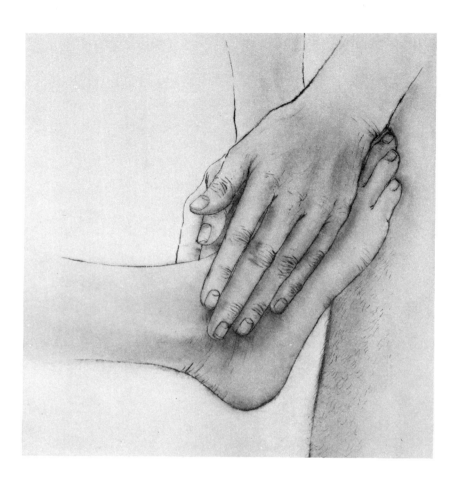

anklebone boogie   ☐ Place the pads of the fingers of both of your hands around the outside edge of the anklebone. Making small circles, just boogie all around the ankle.
☐ (30 seconds).

foot sandwich   ☐ Place the person's foot between the palms of your hands. Using friction, rub the top part of the foot, then the bottom and then both sides at once.
☐ A far-out movement!

Hint: As a finishing tribute to the feet, rub some natural lotion or cream into each foot.

134

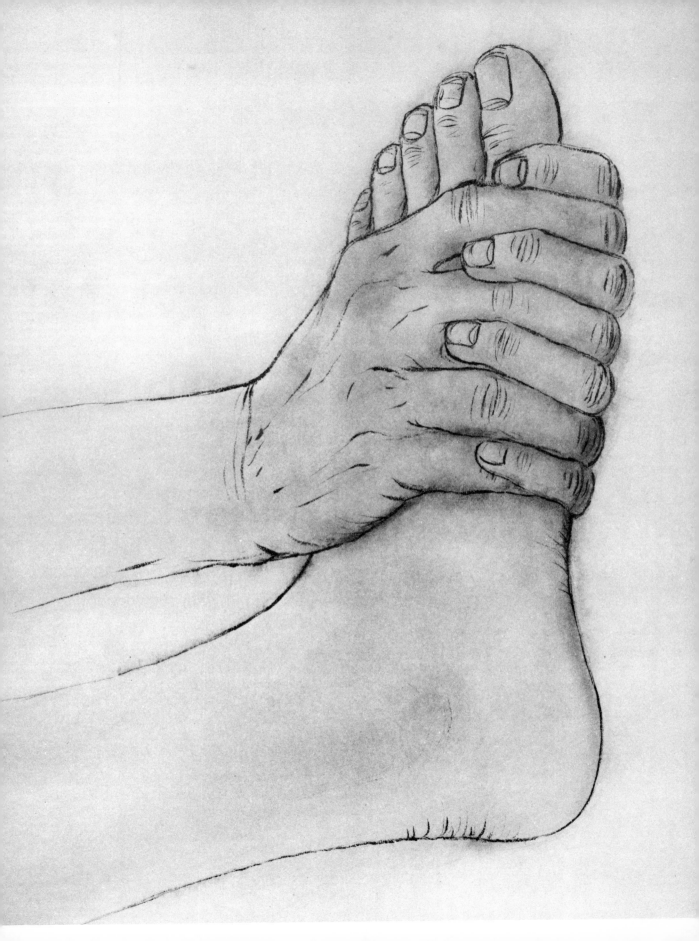

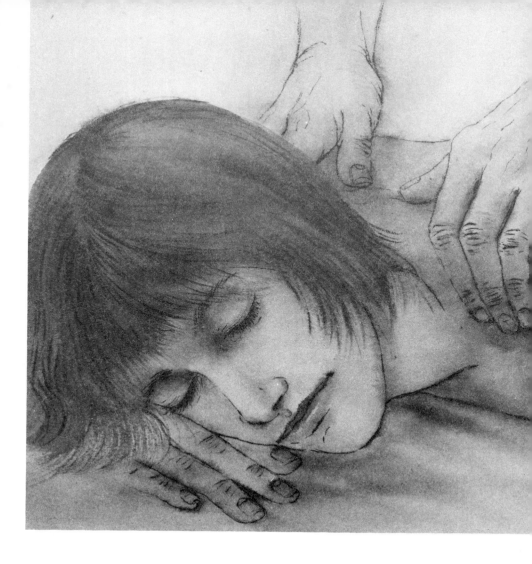

Back   Ask the person to turn over onto the stomach. The arms can be bent beside the head or placed by the sides of the body, whichever is more comfortable.

Hint: Place a rolled-up towel or a small pillow under the upper chest. Do the same thing for under the shins. Do this ONLY if it makes the person more comfortable.

back pressure

☐ Firmly grasp the top of the shoulders with both of your hands. Knead the entire upper back and shoulder areas.
☐ Use medium pressure.
☐ (2 minutes).

136

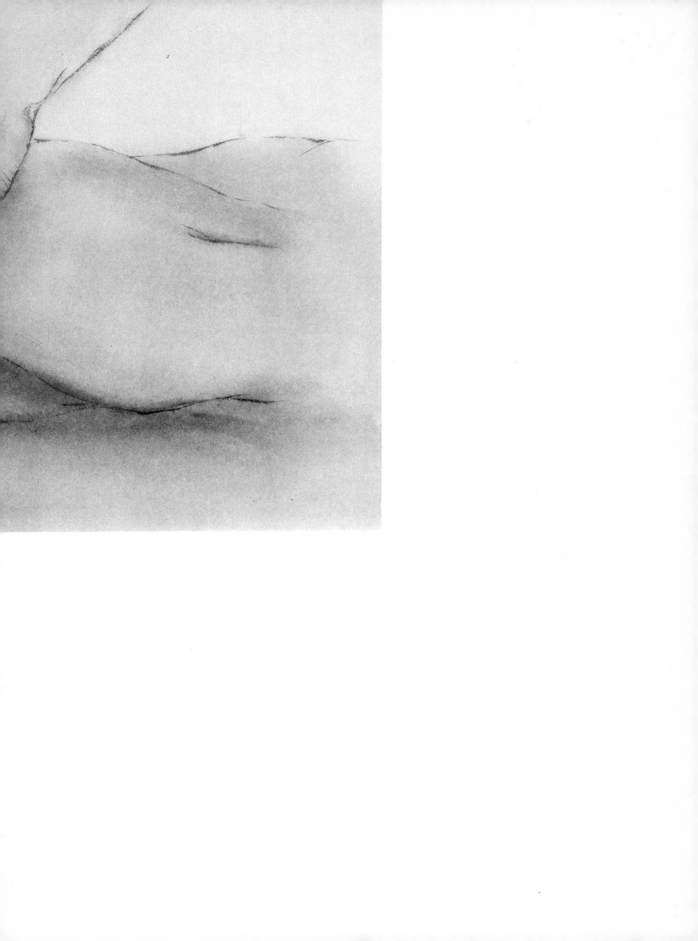

skin flint (petrissage) ☐ Gently pick up the skin of the back between your thumbs and fingers. Squeeze or pinch it gently before letting it drop back into place.
☐ (Do the entire back at least once).

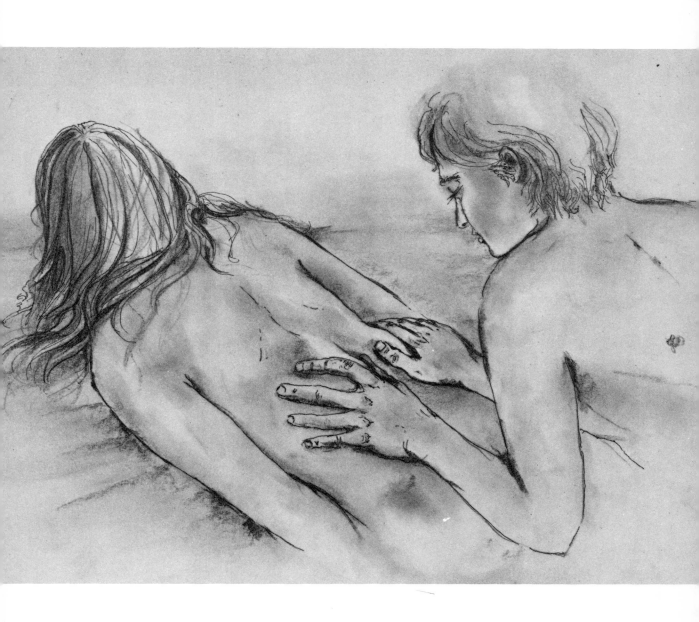

shoulder blade rock   ☐ Destined to reach the top 20 on the Sensation Hit Parade.
☐ Place the palm of one hand over each shoulder blade. Rapidly vibrate the skin back and forth.
☐ Feel the skin slipping and sliding all over the shoulder blades.
☐ (Up to 30 seconds).

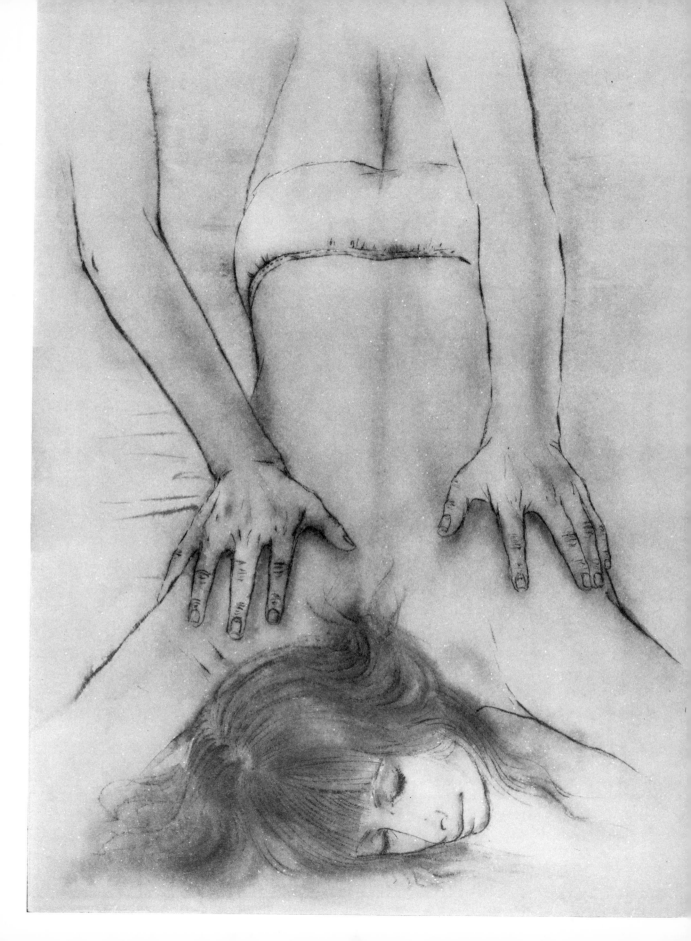

doublecross ☐ This is like making an offer that can't be refused.
☐ Place your hands side by side across the person's lower back. Use friction to pull one of your hands toward you while pushing away with your other hand.
☐ (Go up and down the entire back 3 times).

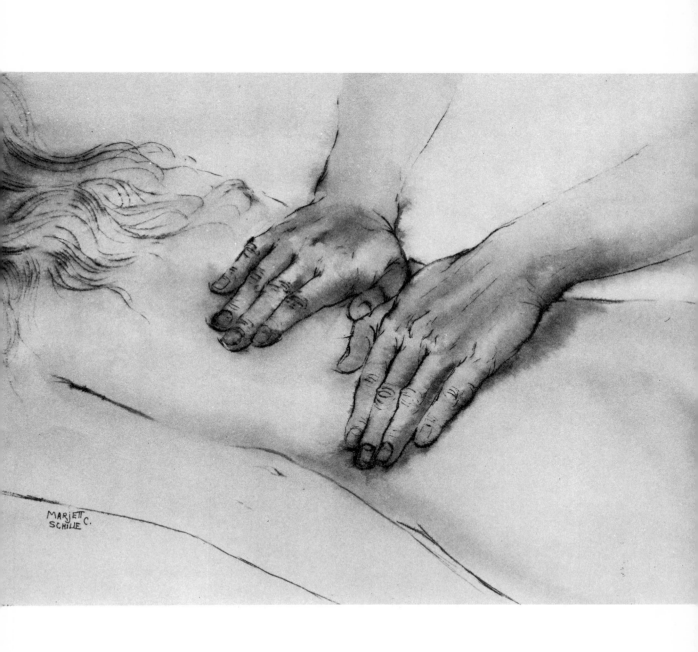

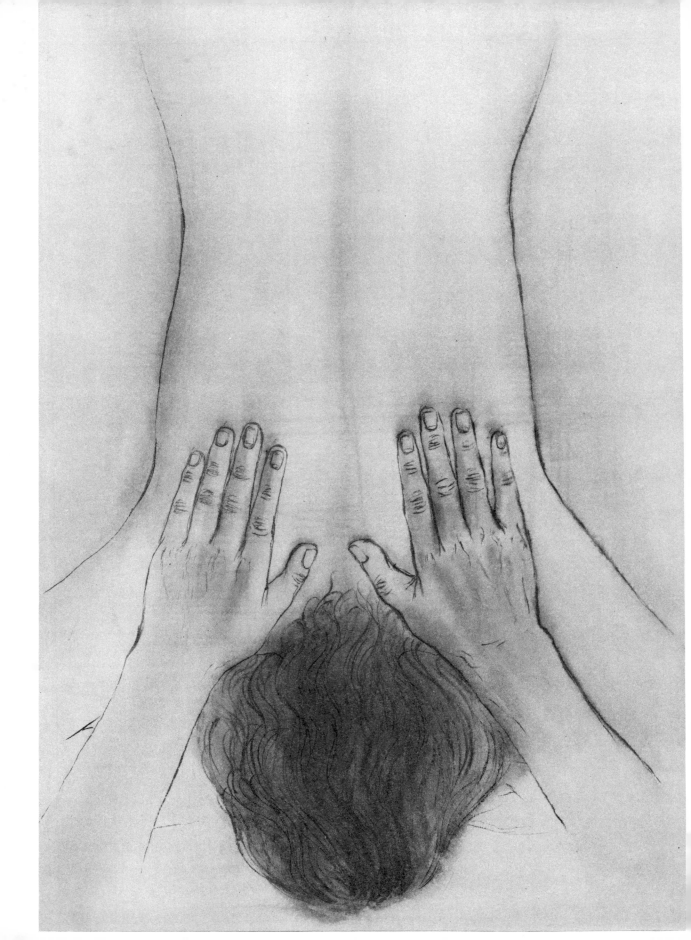

☐ You won't lose faith by doing this one.   **back sliding**
☐ Place both of your hands flat on the person's shoulders.
Use friction to push your hands away from you until they
reach the person's waist. Ease up on the friction as you
lightly return to the shoulders.
☐ (Repeat this stroking movement 4 times).
☐ You can also perform this movement with your hands
going in the opposite direction.

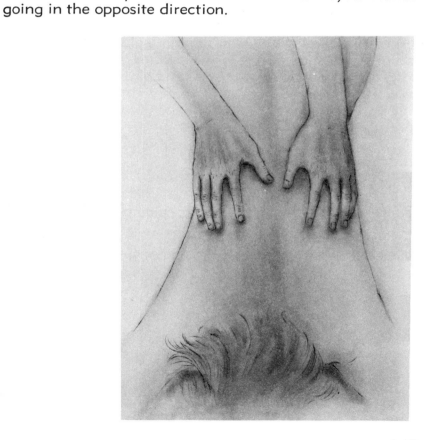

back track   ☐ Keeping your hands flat, stroke the spinal column starting at the base of the neck and alternating your right and left hands.
☐ Use light pressure and rapid, smooth strokes.
☐ This movement relaxes the spinal nerve endings.
☐ (10 strokes with each hand for a total of 20).

vertebra walk   ☐ Spread your first two fingers apart and place one finger on each side of the person's spinal column. Start at the point where the neck joins the shoulders.
☐ Take a walk down to the tail end of the spine. Another variation is to use friction and pull your two fingers from the base of the neck to the tailbone. Use light to medium pressure.
☐ Once you have reached the tailbone, walk back up to the neck.
☐ (2 complete walks).

Hint: For a different sensation try massaging the person's entire back through a soft, thick Turkish towel.

146

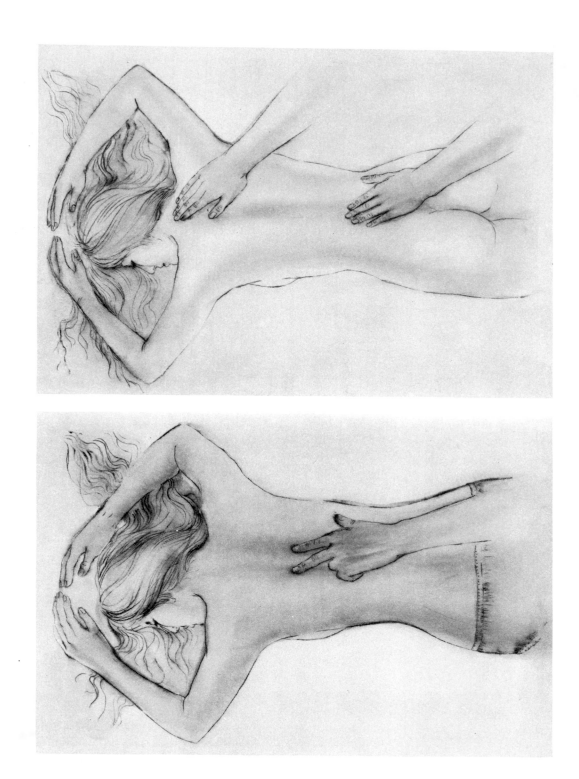

Buttocks

a handful of dough   ☐ Dig in with both hands. Use heavy pressure and knead all over the buttocks.
☐ Feels mighty good.
☐ (1–2 minutes).

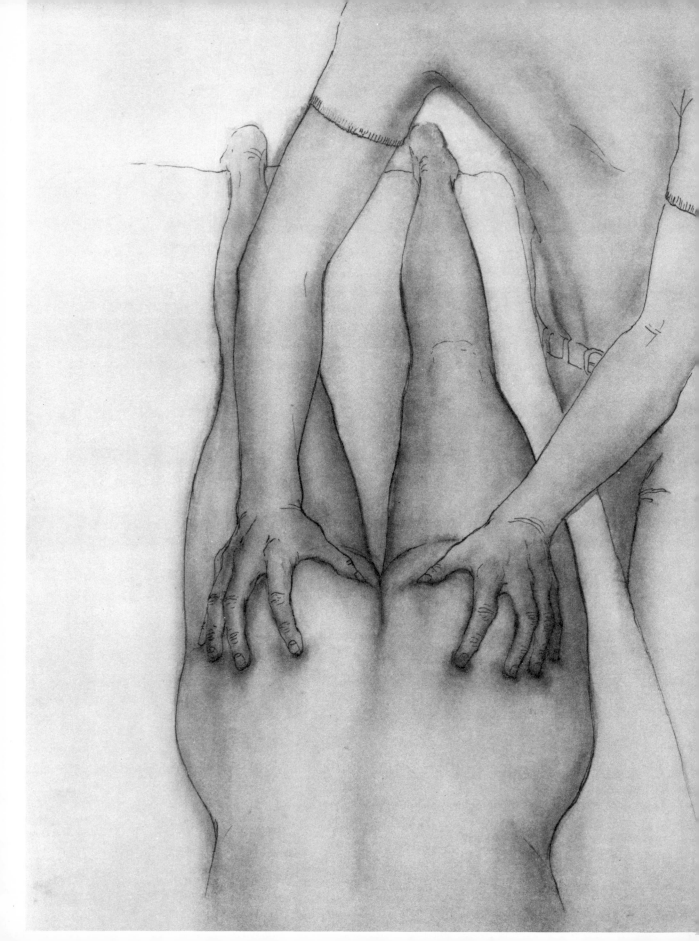

cheek to cheek □ Place your palms flat on the top of the person's buttocks. Rapidly and vigorously shake and vibrate the daylights out of all of those tight-assed stored-up feelings. □ Shake 'em good, they won't fall off. □ (Up to 30 seconds).

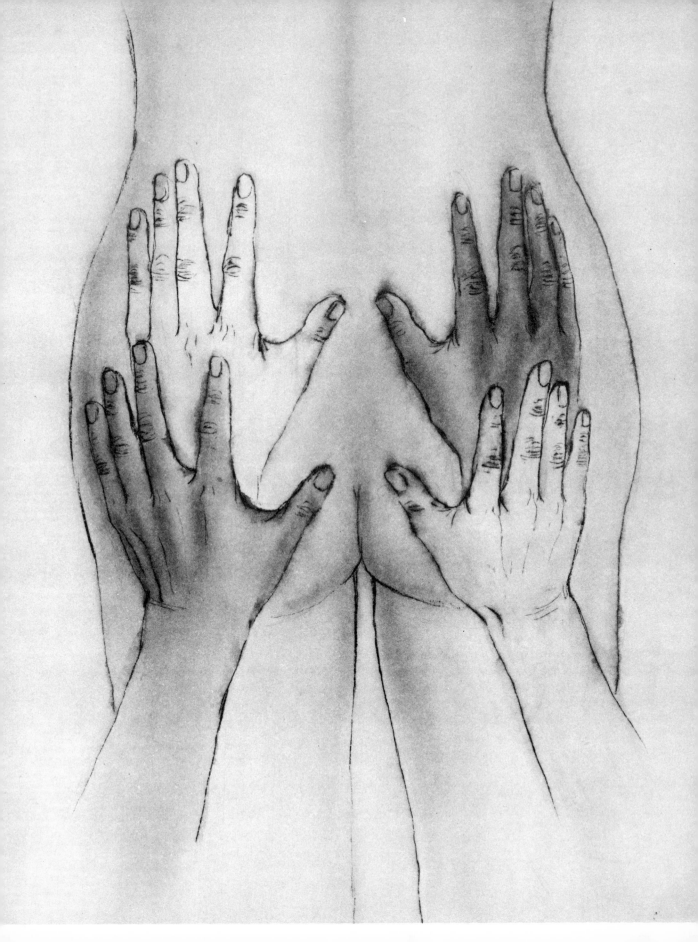

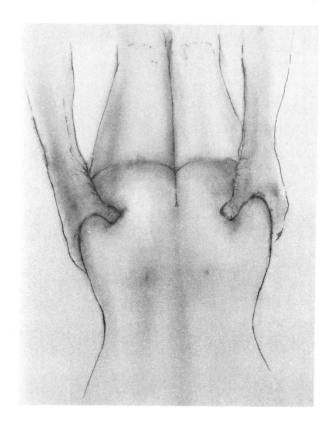

acupressure ☐ A close cousin to acupuncture, except you use the pads of your thumbs instead of needles to stimulate the nerve centers.
☐ Using your thumbs, push in and make deep indentations in the skin, and hold for a few seconds. Move all over the top and sides of the buttocks.
☐ Works wonders.

Backs of Legs

back thigh kneading ☐ Similar to the FRONT THIGH KNEADING movement, page 116. This time you are on the other side of the person's leg.
☐ Mold your hands to fit around the lower thigh just above the knee. Work up an inch at a time to the buttocks.
☐ Use medium-heavy pressure.
☐ Each time you return to the knee, move the position of your hands slightly and work up and back again.
☐ (4 times).

152

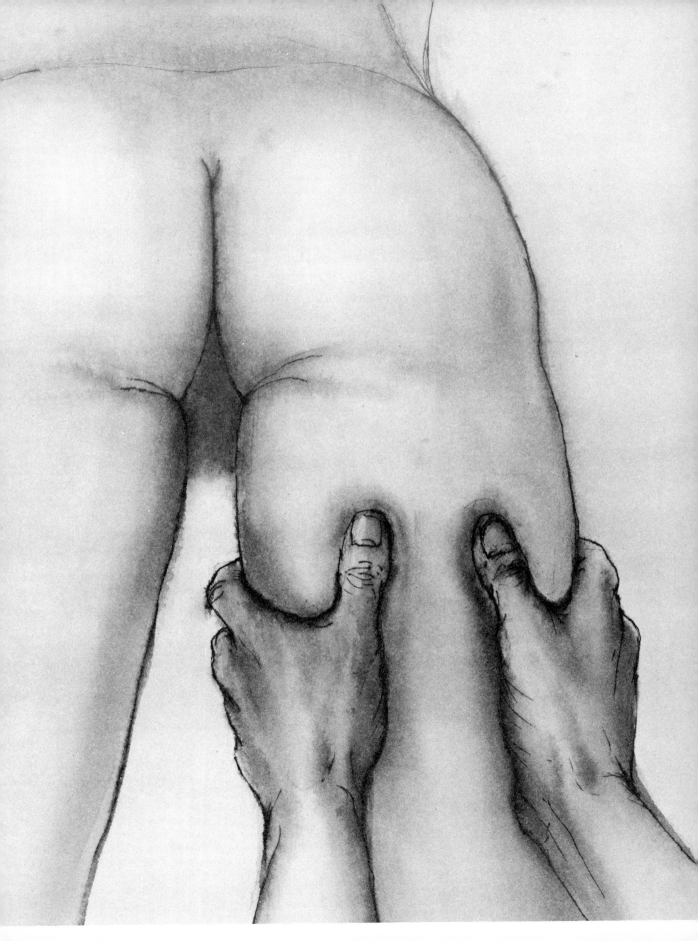

back calf kneading   ☐ Similar to the CALF KNEADING movement, page 112, except the person is now lying on the stomach.
☐ Raise the lower half of the leg off the table. Grasp the calf of the leg about 6 inches above the ankle using both your hands. Work back and forth between the knee and the ankle.
☐ Use medium pressure.
☐ (4 times).

☐ Return the leg to the table or floor when finished with this movement.
Caution: Do not knead directly under the knee.

leg toothpaste squeeze   ☐ Similar to the HAND TOOTHPASTE SQUEEZE movement, page 94. This time you are doing the entire length of the person's leg and ending up at the tips of the toes.
☐ Use medium pressure.
☐ Use a few extra drops of oil if the person has a lot of hair on his or her legs.
☐ (1–2 times, very slowly).

154

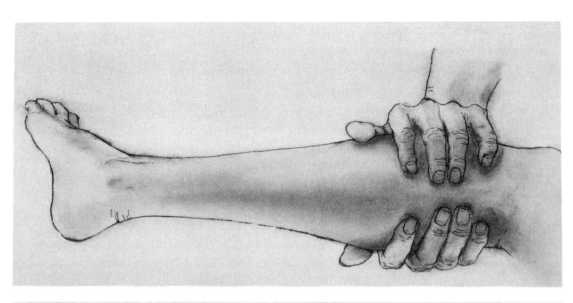

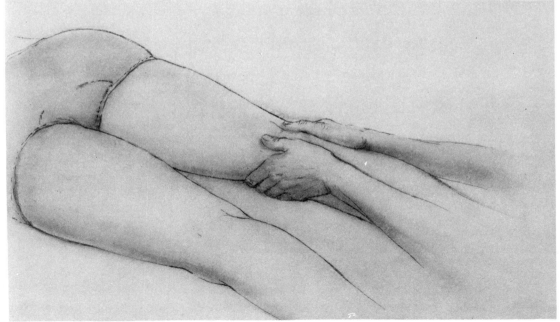

The Finishing Touches

hacking
- ☐ Make both of your hands into the shape of a knife.
- ☐ Keeping your fingers spread apart, with the edge of your hands go ratty-tat-tatty all over the entire back surface of the body. You should feel and hear a FLAT clump-clump sound.
- ☐ (2 times over entire body).

tapping
- ☐ Make your hands into the shape of a garden rake.
- ☐ Use your fingertips to go tippity-tappity all over the entire back part of the body. You should feel and hear a DULL thump-thump sound.
- ☐ Don't forget the soles of the feet.
- ☐ (2 times over entire body).

Caution: Do not strike or hit the kidney area (the soft area on the back just below the last rib) while performing the tapping, hacking, cupping or slapping movements.

156

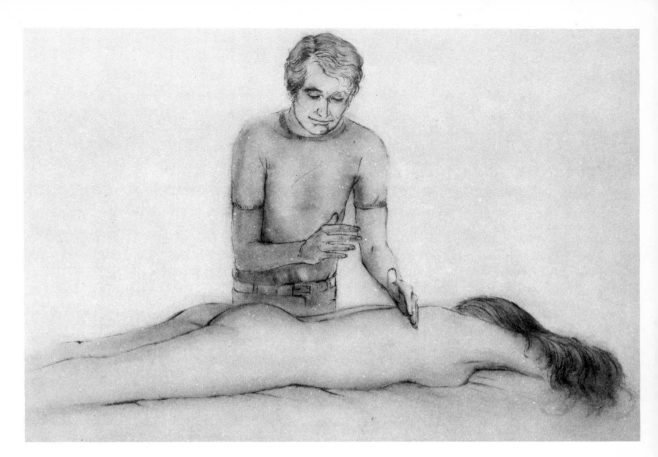

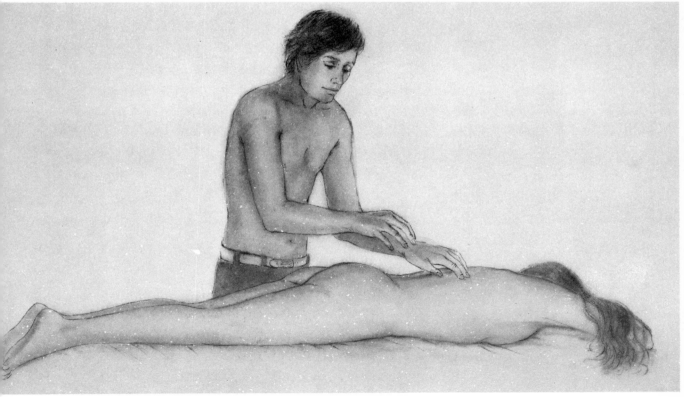

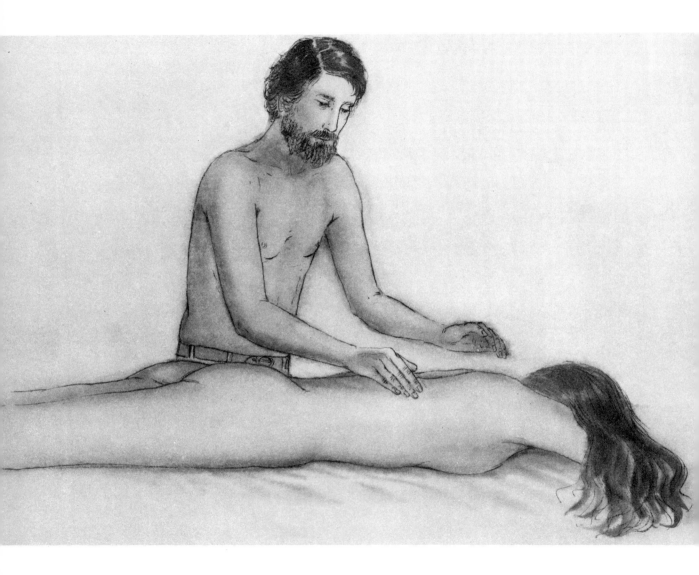

cupping □ Make your hands into the shape of a seashell.
□ Go clop-clopping all over the entire back surface of the body. You should feel and hear a HOLLOW whop-whop sound.
□ (2 times over entire body).

158

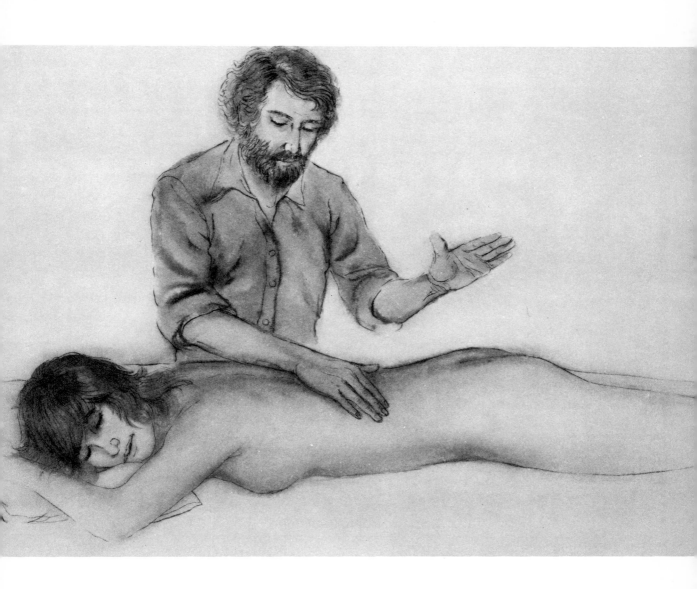

☐ Make your hands flat like a pancake.   **slapping**
☐ Go on a gentle spanking tour all over the entire back
surface of the body. You should feel and hear a slightly
SHARP smack-smack sound.
☐ (2 times over entire body).

159

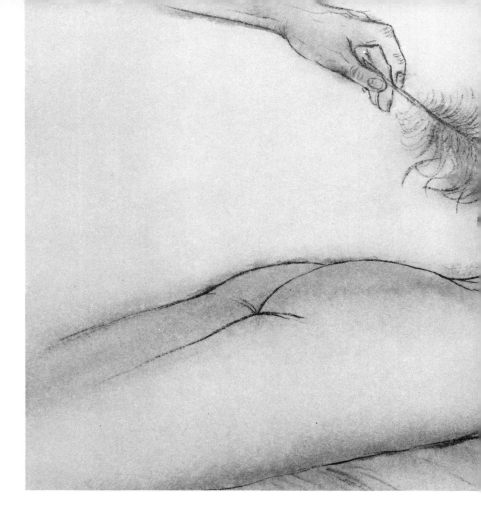

**The Icing
on the Cake** These next movements are guaranteed to win friends and influence people.

raking ☐ You'll dig gardening after this one.
☐ Make both of your hands into the shape of a garden rake. Ever so lightly drag the rakes all over the entire back surface of your friend's body.

Hint: You can use your palms if the person is ticklish.
☐ (Continue for as long as you both wish).

feathering

☐ This is like the touch of the gods. A large, billowy ostrich feather works best.
☐ Go over the entire back surface of your friend's body.
☐ (Again, time is not important).

160

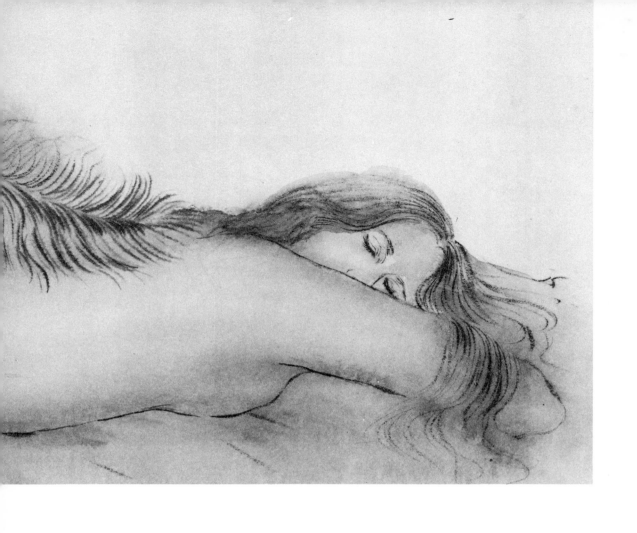

silk king ☐ Same game, except use a lightweight silk scarf this time.

fur out ☐ Use a piece of fur this time.

hair raising ☐ If you happen to have long hair, try dragging your hair all over your friend's body.
☐ Absolutely DY-NO-MITE!

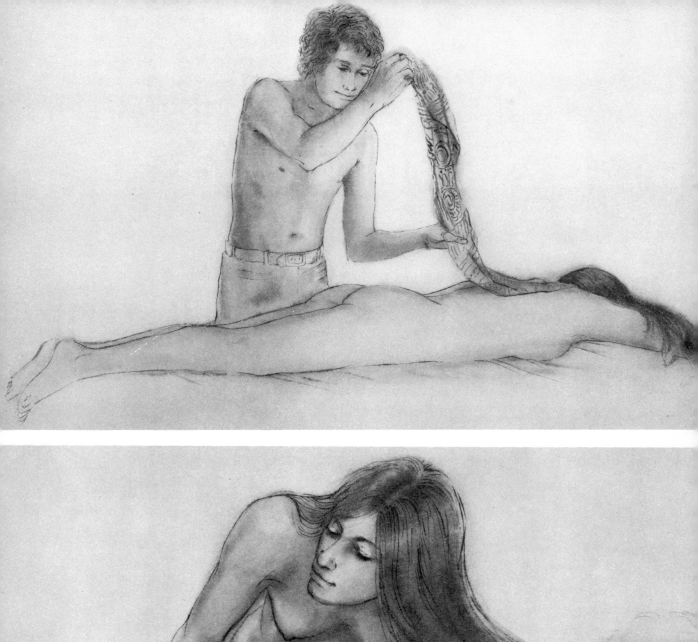
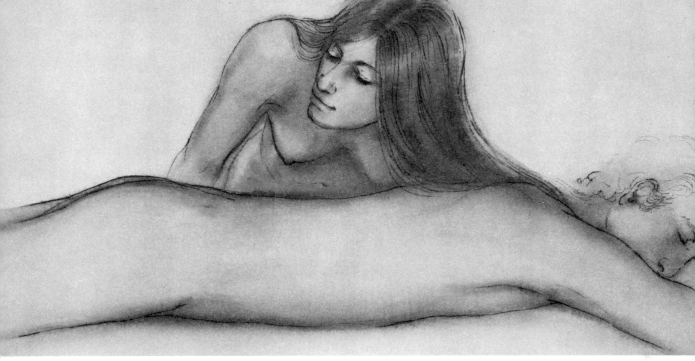

mind blowing ☐ Another Oscar Award–winning finish.
☐ Hold your mouth about 2 inches from your friend's body and gently blow all over the entire surface of the body.

The Final Touch ☐ This is the very last movement and it is an energy exchanger.
☐ Rub your hands together briskly until nice and warm. Then hold your hands with one hand BARELY touching the surface of the back of your friend's neck and the other hand BARELY touching the surface of the lower back.
☐ Your hands should just barely touch the surface of the person's skin. It is like trying to feel the fuzz on a ripe peach.
☐ Keep your hands motionless in this position for 1–2 minutes. While your hands are in this position, plant the following suggestion in the mind of your friend:
You feel much more relaxed now.
You feel happier and more aware.
Next time you will relax more easily
and enjoy the sensations
from my touch even more.
☐ Now gently remove both of your hands at once and remain silent for a few minutes.

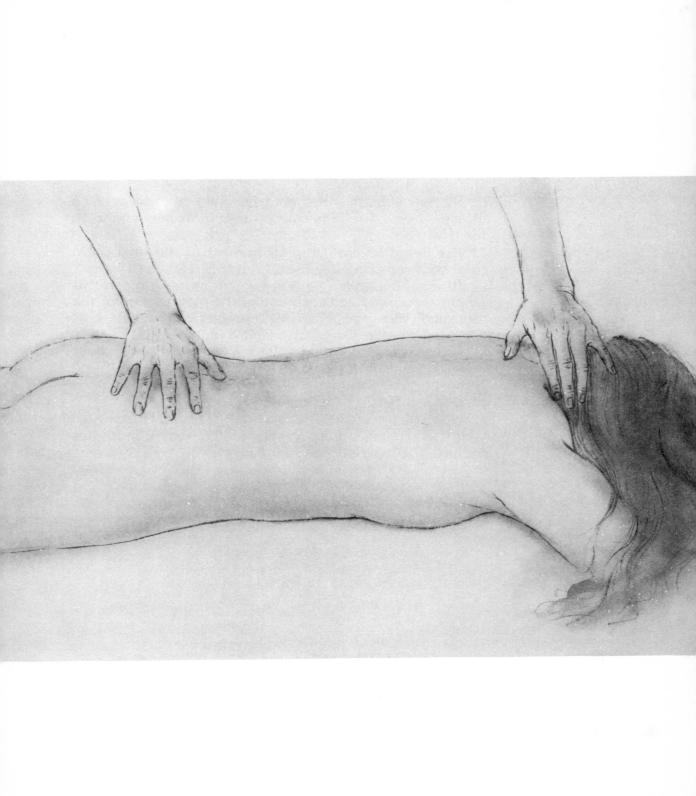

☐ Congratulations!

☐ By now your friend should be quite relaxed or even asleep. If your friend is asleep, let him or her remain so for a while.

☐ I've heard several people comment at the finish of a total body massage, "I haven't felt this relaxed in years."

☐ It may have taken you an hour or more to reach this point if you practiced each one of the movements for the total body massage. The time, however, will decrease as you become more adept at giving a massage.

☐ After several practice sessions it should take about 30–40 minutes to complete a total body massage. If you complete the massage in 15 minutes, you are going too fast. It is difficult to go too slowly.

☐ Now you are anxiously awaiting your turn. Do not rush your friend to get started on you. Wait at least 15 minutes or until another time for your turn.

Hint: When you feel comfortable and proficient at giving a total body massage, try giving an entire massage with your eyes closed. A very touching experience.

THREE
MASSAGING A CHILD

Life is a flame that is always burning itself out.
But it catches fire again every time a child is born.
George Bernard Shaw

Kids love to be massaged. Have you ever noticed how often small children touch each other? Touching, rubbing and physical contact with parents, other children and grownups are quite common during a child's early years. Regrettably, touching behavior becomes less frequent, and in many cases nonexistent, as a child grows up.

☐ One of the main problems between parents and children, especially when the son or daughter is a teenager, is the loss of COMMUNICATION and AFFECTION. Words help, but touch is essential to maintaining a lasting bond. Massaging your children, whatever their ages may be, is putting LOVE and CARE into them.

☐ Ashley Montagu, a famous anthropologist, made a powerful statement in his book TOUCHING:

It has been remarked that in the final analysis
every tragedy is a failure in communication.
And what the child receiving inadequate cutaneous
    (touching) stimulation
suffers from is the failure of
integrative development as a human being,
a failure in the communication
of the fact that he is being loved.
By being stroked, and caressed,
and carried, and cuddled, and cooed to,
by being loved, he learns to stroke
and caress and cuddle, and coo to and love others.
In this sense love is sexual
in the healthiest sense of that word.
It implies involvement, concern,
responsibility, tenderness, and awareness
of the needs and vulnerabilities of the other.

168

☐ Parents get uptight because of their children; children get uptight because of their parents. They literally get out of touch, and keep at arm's distance and lose the human touch.

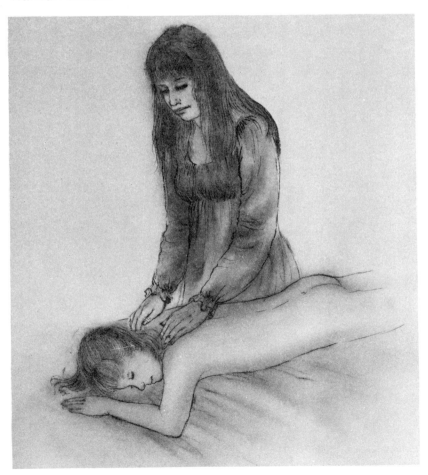

☐ When massaging a child you can use any or all of the movements in Section Two, A TOTAL BODY MASSAGE. Lots of long, gentle, stroking motions seem to be a big hit. Do not use heavy pressure or force a child to stay still for an entire massage.

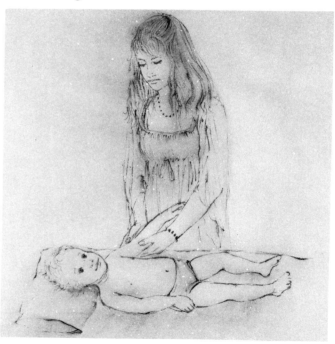

☐ Massage is also a good way to relax an overtired or hyperactive child.
☐ With babies and younger children, stick to gentle stroking and patting movements only.
☐ Massage your children regularly and they will grow to enjoy it and their lives with you more fully.

170

FOUR
MASSAGING YOURSELF

If you do not get it from yourself
Where will you go for it?
                    Old Zen Poem

A self-massage serves a good purpose even though it isn't as satisfying as a two-way massage. You can massage yourself anytime you feel the need. A little self-massage in the morning better prepares you to cope with the upcoming events of the day. After work it helps you to unwind tension from your mind and body. At the end of the day it paves the way to a restful sleep.

☐ First, take off all clothing and jewelry. A warm shower, bath or sauna beforehand will help you to relax. Sit down in a comfortable position on a bed or on the floor. A bed is okay when giving yourself a massage.

☐ You may perform most of the movements shown in Section Two, A TOTAL BODY MASSAGE. The exceptions, of course, are movements for the back, which is difficult to reach.

☐ While sitting up, do your head, face, neck, shoulders, hands, arms, thighs, lower legs and feet. Put special emphasis on the face, neck, hands and feet.

☐ You can massage your shoulders by crisscrossing your arms and applying a kneading action, using your thumbs and fingers.

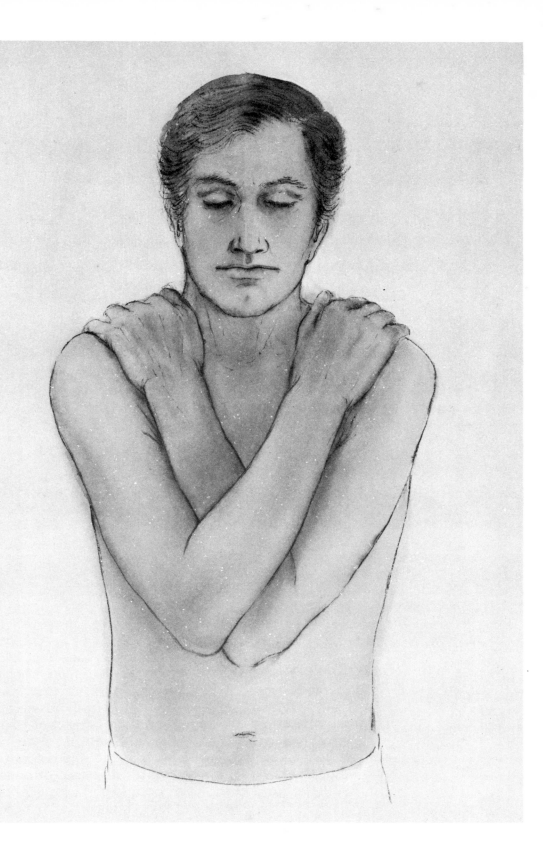

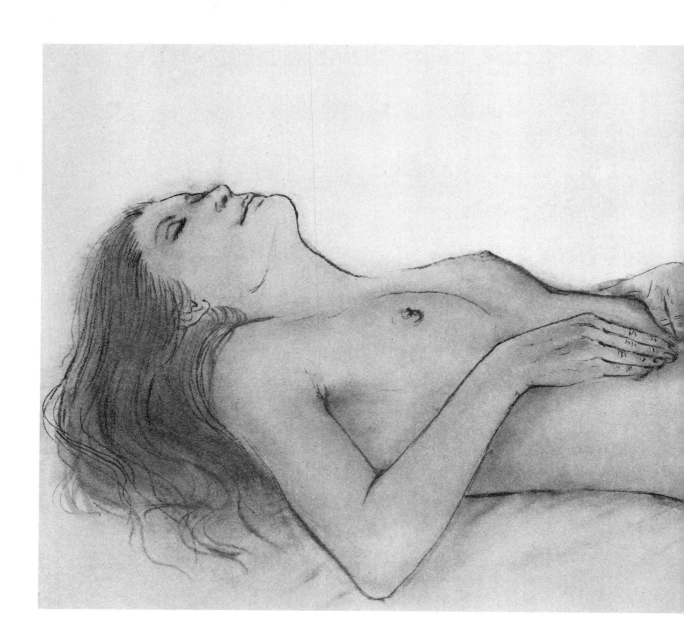

☐ Now lie down. Arch your legs and place the soles of both feet flat on the bed or floor. Massage your chest and abdominal area.

☐ For the finishing touches, stand up and massage your buttocks and slap everywhere on your body that you can comfortably reach. Then shake and vibrate your arms, hands, legs—let your entire body shake like a bowlful of Jell-O or like a skeleton rattling all its bones at once.

☐ Really let go and shake it, baby—you won't break.

174

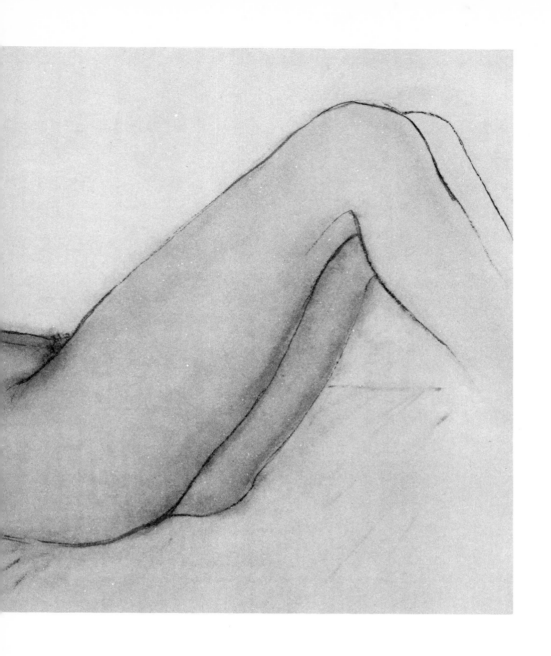

SELF-MASSAGE FOR THE FIVE MOST COMMON EVERYDAY PHYSICAL ACHES AND PAINS

One:
Headache

Most headaches are the result of too much muscular tension. What caused the tension in the first place is another matter. Before reaching for the aspirin bottle or other medication, try the following self-remedy.

Place the first three fingers of each hand
on your neck at the base of your skull.
With firm pressure,
make tiny circular movements on this area
or do the NECK VIBRATION, page 75,
(no longer than 3 minutes).

176

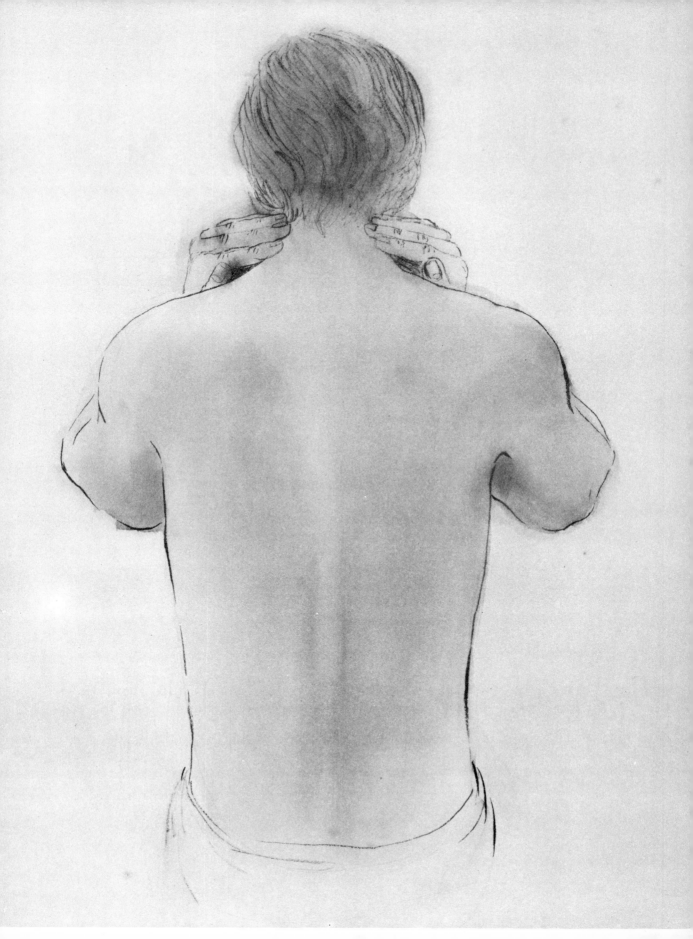

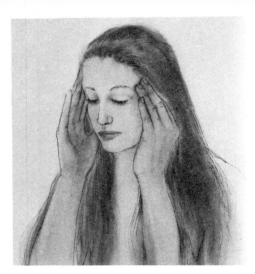

Massage around your temples for a couple of minutes.

Rotate your head slowly in a circle, going clockwise.
Then reverse the direction (counterclockwise).
Do this movement several times.
Turn your head slowly from side to side
as far as you can each time.

This next massage movement may seem silly to you
but it often works!
Perform deep kneading with the top of your thumb
all over your big toe and the one next to it.
Massage the area on the foot
just below these two toes.
I won't go into details about why this helps
but will just mention that it is related
to acupuncture techniques developed by the Chinese.

Stand up and make your body shake all over.

☐ If you still have the headache at this point, tie a towel securely around your head and massage the top and sides of your head through the towel.

Almost everyone has some daily tension in these areas.
□ Get yourself into a comfortable sitting position on a bed or the floor. For a self-massage of the neck, perform the following movements:

Neck spiral, page 73.
Neck vibration, pages 74 and 75.

□ For a self-massage of the shoulders, perform the following movements:

Shoulder crisscross, page 173.
(This is similar to
the Piano Roll Blues movement,
page 77.)
Shoulder squeeze, page 78.
Crisscross your arms
while doing this one.
Shoulder rotation, page 80.

□ For a self-massage of the back, reach around and perform kneading movements on all the areas of your back that you can comfortably reach. Perform rubbing movements on both upper and lower back. You can lie on the floor and by moving up and down and sideways cause the skin to slide over the muscles and bones of your back.

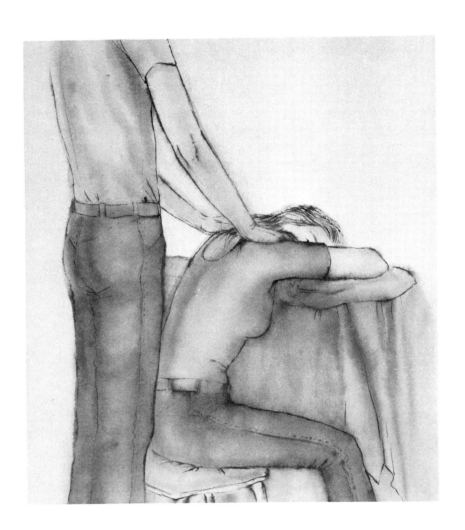

☐ If you have someone available to give you a quick back massage, the best position for receiving it is sitting at the end of a table with your arms and head resting comfortably on two or three pillows located near the edge. This position is better than lying down since the neck, shoulder and back muscles are looser and more relaxed.

180

□ You can have your friend work on your neck, shoulders and back, doing the movements for those areas as shown in Section Two.

Lie flat on your back with your legs flexed, knees bent and feet flat on the bed or floor. Use the self-massage movement on page 174 and the abdominal area movements on pages 108 to 111.
□ About 3–5 minutes on this area is sufficient. These movements are also excellent for relieving constipation.

Three: Knots in the Stomach or Gut

Start with a hot water and Epsom salts foot bath. Soak feet for about 10 minutes.
□ Now give yourself a nice foot massage, using the movements on pages 126 to 135. Massage your legs, using the movements on pages 112 to 125.

Four: Leg Aches and Cramps—Tired and Burning Feet

□ If you want to apply a good muscle liniment to your feet and legs, use a product called BANALG. It is a mild liniment in a nongreasy base. The main ingredients are menthol and camphor. Also, you may use some plain camphor oil or an oriental product called Tiger Balm.

footnotes

Four days prior to the start of your menstrual period perform the following massage movements on yourself or have someone else do them for you:

Five: Menstrual Cramps

□ Rub around the anklebone.
(See the Anklebone Boogie, page 134.)

181

□ Pay particular attention to the area between the anklebone and the heel.
□ Do a little deep digging with the tip of the thumb.
□ Massage this whole area for about 3 minutes.
□ Lie flat on your back, with knees bent, legs flexed and feet flat on the table or floor, and do the abdominal movements on pages 108 to 111.

Massage During Pregnancy

□ A total body massage is relaxing and reassuring to an expectant mother. It will help make the birth process a more positive and less traumatic experience for both mother and child. If you are planning on having children, I recommend that you read the excellent book BIRTH WITHOUT VIOLENCE by Frederick Leboyer, a compassionate French physician. Dr. Leboyer attempts to make the infant's entry into this world as gentle and non-traumatic as possible. Since breathing will begin naturally, he does not believe in spanking the newborn. Lights and noise in the delivery room are kept to a minimum. Both the mother and the doctor gently massage the newborn for five minutes while the infant rests in a fetal position on top of the mother's abdomen.
□ The importance of touch in infancy cannot be overemphasized. James Prescott, a developmental neuropsychologist at the National Institute of Child Health and Human Development, believes that violence, alcohol and drug problems originate in infancy due to the lack of touching and body contact with the mother.

Caution: Do not massage the abdominal or uterus area during pregnancy. Soft stroking movements, however, are good right up to the time of delivery.

FIVE
AN EROTIC MASSAGE

That's all there is
When you do it with love.
                              Anonymous

A stimulating erotic massage can follow a total body massage or it can be done alone.

☐ Erotic massage can be thought of as extended foreplay. It produces relaxed stimulation and tremendously enhances the joy of sex.

☐ The sexually sensual touch is not something you do to someone, or for someone, but with someone.

☐ And now, lovers of the world, you are ready to pleasure each other.

moon talk ☐ Use your forefinger to lightly trace a quarter-moon crescent around the heel of your lover's hand.

☐ Very lightly make a one-finger oval pattern on the inside of the wrist.

☐ (There are no time restrictions for any of the movements in the EROTIC MASSAGE section.)

184

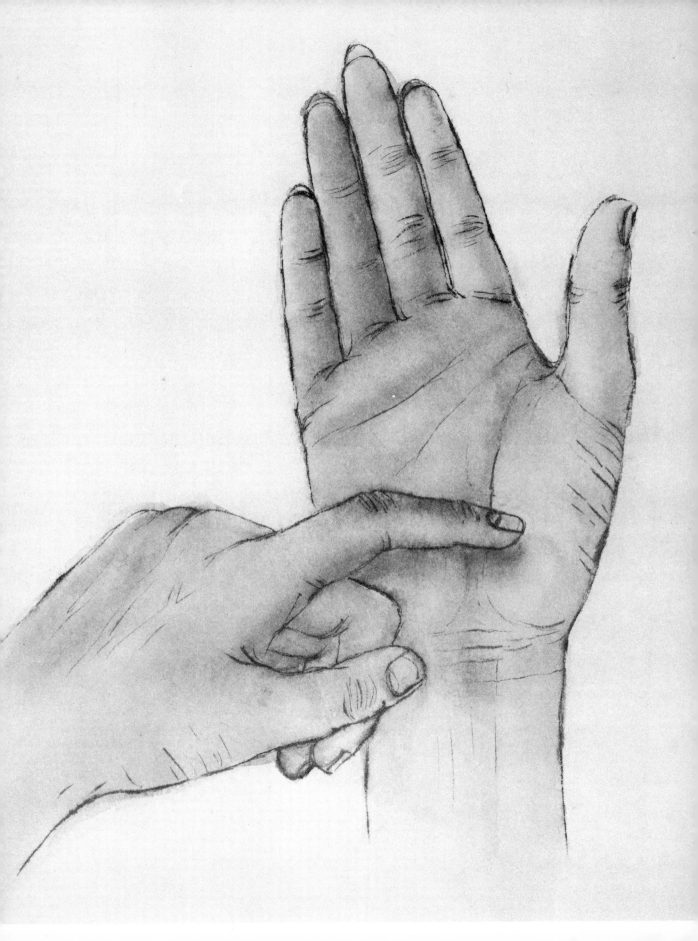

ear- ☐ This movement is ear-resistible.
resistible ☐ Use your first two fingers to lightly trace around the outer ear, inside the ear and on the earlobe.

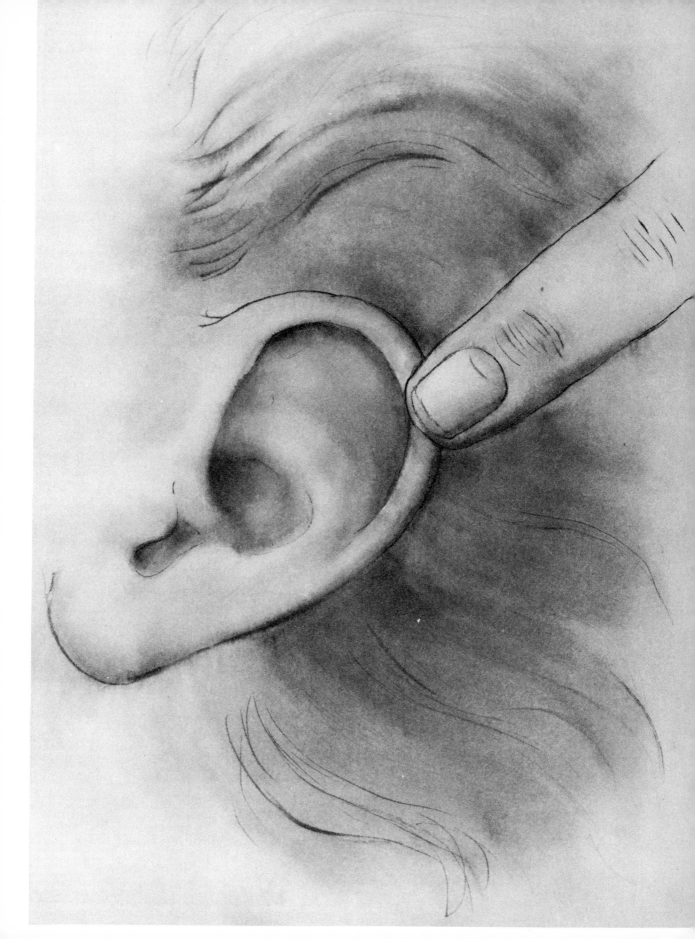

**footing
it** □ Use the fingers to lightly stroke all over the feet and between the toes.

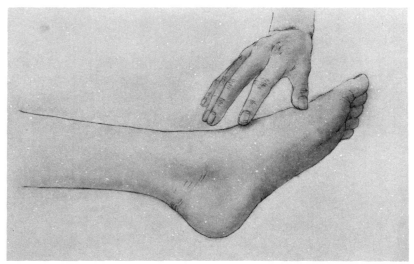

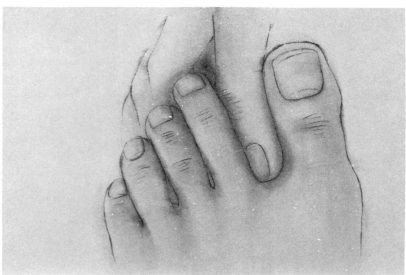

☐ Rub around the ankle and heel area.

☐ Similar to the ANKLEBONE BOOGIE movement, page 134, this movement stimulates nerve endings connected to the sexual organs.

ankle/heel turn-on

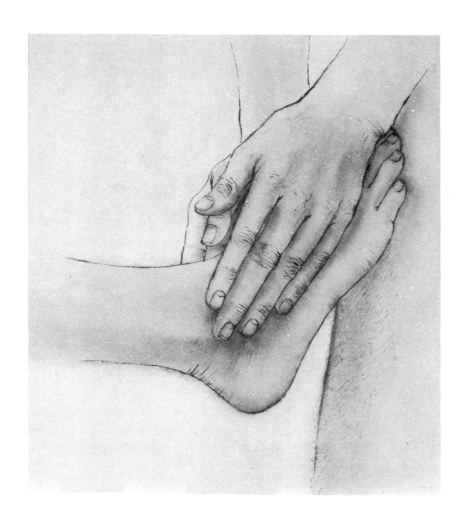

french ☐ Slowly and gently rake the fingertips of one of your
tickle hands all over your lover's body.

lip trace ☐ Lightly, like a butterfly, do a one-finger trace on the
surface of your lover's lips.

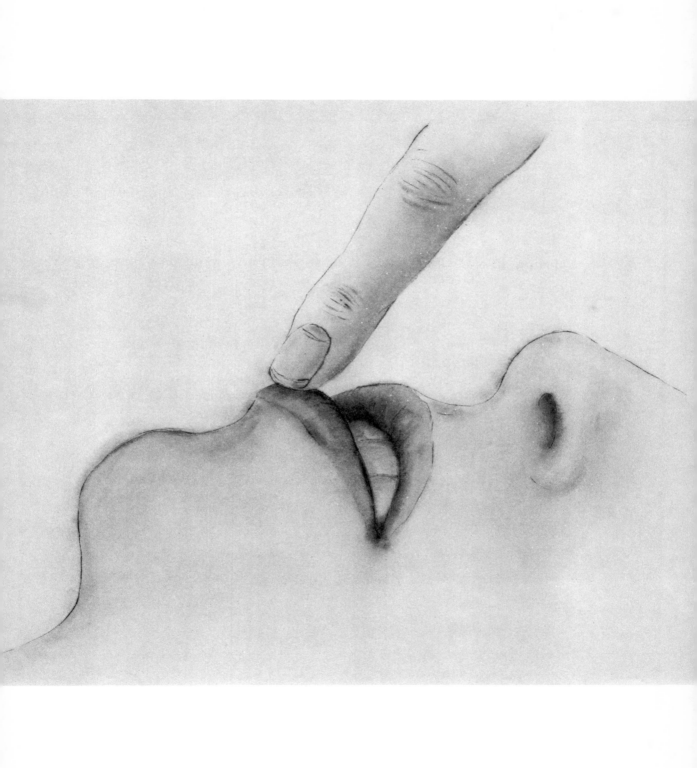

breast figure-8 ☐ Use your forefinger to make figure-8 patterns all over the breast area, occasionally brushing the nipple like a bee landing on a fresh honey-laden Blue Appolusa flower.

closing in ☐ Light, one-finger stroking on the inside of the thighs is delicious.

silky touch ☐ Take a lightweight silk scarf and drag it all over your lover's body. Slowly, sensually trail it over the genital area.
☐ Spread the legs and very slowly and ever-so-lightly trace the scarf through this highly sensitive area. Keep the other hand on your lover's body.

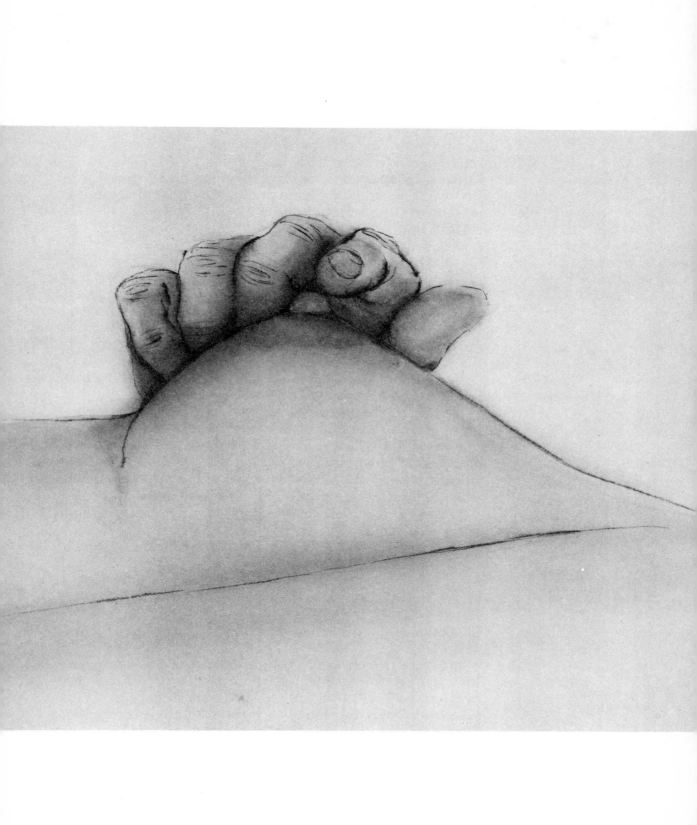

☐ A soft piece of fur or a large billowy feather works wonders.

☐ Softly blowing air, taking nibbly-sized bites or moistly tonguing all over the body is superb.

☐ To massage his penis and surrounding area use the first two fingers of one hand and lightly make tiny circles underneath the scrotum and on the testicles.

☐ Run both of your fingers in a soft stroking action up and down the shaft of his penis.

☐ Moisten both of your fingers with some saliva or cream and trace around and directly on the head of his penis.

☐ There are several ways to massage her vagina and the surrounding area. First, use one of your fingers to lightly make small circles on the area between the bottom of the vagina and the anal opening.

☐ Occasionally, a couple of quick light strokes on the anus feels erotic to many women.

☐ Spread apart the first two fingers of your hand and lightly trace up and down the outer lips of her vagina.

☐ Take the forefinger of one hand and gently pull back on the skin hood covering the clitoris. Moisten the forefinger of the other hand with saliva or cream. Now make tiny circles around and on her clitoral head. If massaging the clitoris directly is too sensitive, then stroke it tenderly with the skin covering in place.

☐ Insert one or two fingers into her vagina and massage around the inside walls.

☐ There is no particular right way to stimulate the genitals. Use your own imagination, find out what feels best to your lover and DO IT!

☐ You are now on your own.

Hint: Here is a unique sensual experience you and your lover can try sometime. Spend part of a day with your eyes closed and have your lover lead you around, feed you, bathe you and make love to you before reopening your eyes. A gratifying experience.

194

SIX
A GROUP MASSAGE

Now join your hands, and with your hands your hearts.
William Shakespeare

A massage by two or more people is a unique and satisfying experience. It is best to use combinations of two-on-one or four-on-one. This is preferable to three-on-one or five-on-one since the movements are counterbalanced when using an even number of people on each side.

TWO-ON-ONE One person can massage the face while the other is working on the stomach. Next, with one person on each side, use smooth, rhythmic and coordinated movements going from the chest all the way down to the feet. Perform the movements shown in Section Two, A TOTAL BODY MASSAGE.
☐ Here is the order for doing the front of the person lying down:

Chest
Hands
Arms
Front of Legs and Thighs
Ankles
Feet

☐ When you finish with the feet, help the person roll over onto the stomach.
☐ Continue with:

Shoulders
Back
Buttocks
Back of Thighs and Legs

196

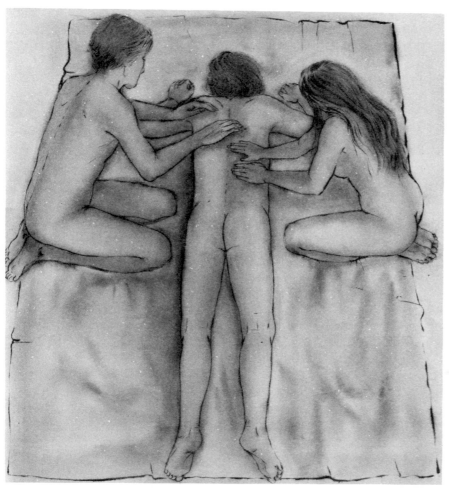

☐ Now for the finish strokes. One of you can work on the upper body—shoulders, back, hands and arms. The other can work on the lower body—buttocks, thighs, legs and feet.

197

FOUR-ON-ONE Four people massaging another person is the limit for a comfortable massage. With six or more people you will get in each other's way.

☐ Begin with each of you working on one of these areas:

First person	Face
Second person	Stomach and Chest
Third person	Right Foot
Fourth person	Left Foot

☐ Finish the above areas together and move on to:

First person	Left Hand and Arm
Second person	Right Hand and Arm
Third person	Right Ankle, Lower Leg and Thigh
Fourth person	Left Ankle, Lower Leg and Thigh

☐ All together now, gently roll the person over onto the stomach. And carry on:

First person	Left side of Shoulder, Back and Buttock
Second person	Right side of Shoulder, Back and Buttock
Third person	Back of Right Thigh and Leg
Fourth person	Back of Left Thigh and Leg

☐ Work on these same areas when performing the FINISHING STROKES.

☐ Now place your hands in the following manner:

First person	One hand on the Left side of the Back and the other hand on the Left Buttock
Second person	One hand on the Right side of the Back and the other hand on the Right Buttock
Third person	One hand on the Right Thigh and the other hand on the Right Leg
Fourth person	One hand on the Left Thigh and the other on the Left Leg

☐ Keep your hands in place for a minute or two and allow the good will to soak in. Watch each other for a signal and slowly remove all of your hands at the same time.

LIFTING AND ROCKING

This doesn't have to be a part of a massage. It can be done anytime several people are gathered together.
☐ Lifting and rocking is a popular feature of encounter groups. You need at least six or eight people to perform this movement, depending upon the height and weight of the person to be lifted. Be sure to have enough people available so that the person can be lifted without strain.

199

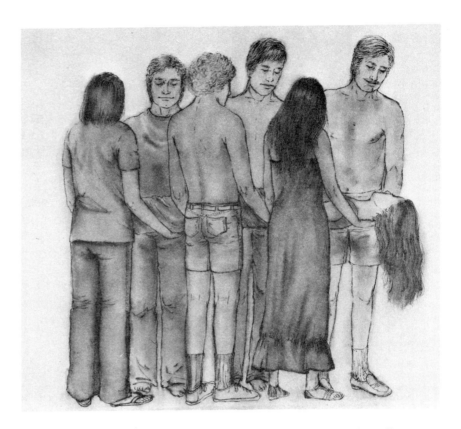

☐ Start with the person lying face up on the floor or ground with eyes closed. Have two or three people stand on each side of the person lying down. If possible, have another person stand behind the person's head. Otherwise, the two people nearest the head can support it by using one hand each. In unison, gently slip the palms of your hands under the body and, very slowly, lift the person to your waist level.

☐ Slowly rock the person back and forth. Do this for

about 3 minutes. If there are enough of you to do it without strain, lift the person up to your face level and then, very slowly, lower him or her to the floor. In unison, slowly remove your hands. Let the person lie still for a few minutes. Take turns.

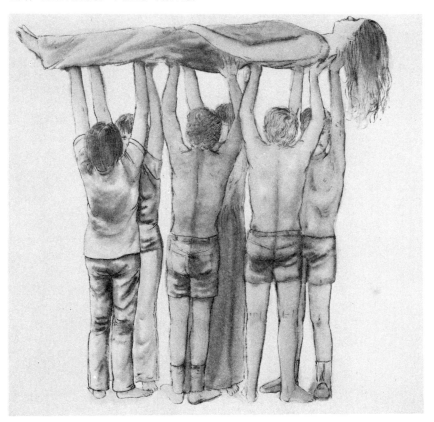

☐ Something everyone should experience at least once in a lifetime.

SEVEN
OTHER CONSIDERATIONS

This section deals with daily personal habits that are essential to your overall HEALTH and HAPPINESS.

STRESS AND NERVOUS TENSION

Nothing in the affairs of men is worthy of great anxiety.
Plato

Considering how lighthearted we feel when we do not take ourselves seriously, it is surprising how difficult the attainment of this sensible and practical attitude seems to be. It is apparently much easier to be serious than frivolous.

Eric Hoffer

We all have some stress in our daily lives. Stress is related to work, family, environment and society.
☐ Dr. Hans Seyle, famous for his lifelong research on stress, states:

The stress of living with one another
still represents
one of the greatest causes of distress.

☐ Some stressors can be thought of as good: working energetically at something you thoroughly enjoy doing, some nervousness before giving a speech, the joy of victory, sheer delight and so on.
☐ Many stressors are bad. They do damage to the body and bring havoc and unpleasantness to the mind. The effects of stress are varied, but generally they mean that we BURN OURSELVES OUT FASTER.
☐ Dr. Seyle points out:

Mental tensions, frustrations, insecurity and aimlessness

are among the most damaging stressors,
and psychosomatic studies have shown
how often they cause migraine headache,
peptic ulcers, heart attacks, hypertension,
mental disease, suicide, or just hopeless unhappiness.
Nothing paralyzes your efficiency more
than frustration;
nothing helps more than success.
But successful activity,
no matter how intense,
leaves you with comparatively few scars;
it causes stress but little,
if any, distress.

He says another big problem area is "the craving for approval and the dread of censure."
☐ Stress, both mental and physical, plays a part in many diseases and unhealthy conditions:

heart attacks	allergies
hypertension	cancer
ulcers	stroke
colitis	alcoholism
nervous disorders	insomnia
colds	depression
headaches	menstrual cramps
hay fever	anxiety attacks
asthma	impotence
backache	frigidity
constipation	eczema
infections	smoking and
diabetes	drug addiction

☐ Even accidents have been shown to be related to preceding stressful events.

☐ Some of the causes of stress are:

Physical factors—heat, cold, pressure (against some part of the body), lack of oxygen, toxic substances, allergies, light, sounds, hunger, injury and sickness.

Psychological factors—money worries, people worries, too many wants, goals that are too high, negative thoughts, indecision, rushing, boredom, too many pressing problems, disorganization, unreasonable expectations of others and trying to manipulate others to do what you want.

These are only some of the major causes of stress.

☐ Let's take a brief look at a sampling of some words in the English language that are associated with stress:

fear	down	low
worry	hate	tired
tension	bitterness	sick
anxiety	jealousy	work
depression	envy	cruelty
problems	loathe	abuse
illness	uptight	dislike
grief	responsibility	grudge
noise	boredom	revenge
hurry	hostility	vindictive
frustration	fatigue	loneliness
strain	overcrowding	ostracize
pressure	rushing	divorce
bad	disorganization	exhaustion
wrong	difficulty	wear
harass	uncontrollable	finances
sad	procrastination	indecision

negative	anguish	fear
tear	disgust	terror
taxes	anger	rage
injury	humiliation	crime
money	guilt	violence
distress		

And, of course, all the gaps—generation, parent-child, men-women, Russian-American-Chinese, political, cultural, energy, environmental, marriage, and on and on and on.

☐ I'm certain you could think of additional words and gaps to add to this list.

In a recent medical book □ the statement was made:

Clinicians estimate that 50–70%
of all the visits to doctors' offices
are for functional illness.
Overutilization of
health-care services for
unsuccessful treatment
of these disorders
is one factor in the
high cost of health care today.

Functional illnesses are those that are directly related to stress of some kind.

☐ In the same book the authors define one of the main manifestations of stress as "bracing." Bracing means a "negative reaction to a stressful event or situation which results in detrimental effects on the body which are manifested in the form of muscular tension or tightening."

□ George B. Whatmore and Daniel R. Kohli, THE PHYSIOPATHOL-OGY AND TREATMENT OF FUNCTIONAL DISORDERS—IN-CLUDING ANXIETY STATES, DEPRESSION AND THE ROLE OF BIOFEEDBACK TRAINING (New York: Grune & Stratton, 1975).

□ One method of reducing stress or "bracing" efforts is to use electronic equipment to help the person recognize the difference between states of stress and states of relaxation. These methods are known by such labels as biofeedback, alpha (brain wave) conditioning, and EMG (muscular) conditioning.

□ Other techniques rely on open discussion and exercises designed to get troublesome things out of the person's system. These techniques have varying degrees of success and are known by such names as Encounter, Human Potential, Self-Actualization, EST, Human Awareness, Bioenergetics and Primal Therapy.

□ One of the best and most inexpensive ways to reduce stress and muscular tension and to promote relaxation is MASSAGE. Let's look at some of the words that denote a few of the feelings and states that result from a good massage:

relaxed	mellow	rejuvenated
caring	loose	friendly
laid back	placid	fun
fulfilled	peaceful	serene
joyful	smiling	alive
passive	asleep	turned on
happy	aware	love
rested	erotic	contented
invigorated	drifting	far out
sensual	self-contained	
floating	trippy	

□ The best way to reduce stress is to eliminate the cause. The second best way, in my opinion, is through the use of a soothing and relaxing total body massage.

208

☐ I'll end this discussion by issuing a brief bit of friendly advice:

Deal with the HERE AND NOW.
The past is gone
and the future is not yet here.
ME is only an instantaneous moment
of your life
at any given time.
Living is NOW,
not yesterday or tomorrow.
And, you pass this way but once.

As William Saroyan once said, "In the time of your life LIVE."

Tell me what you eat,
and I will tell you what you are.
Brillat-Savarin

EATING— FOOD—DIET— WEIGHT CONTROL— NUTRITION

Whatever you may wish to call the process, eating determines to a large extent how you feel mentally and physically.

☐ At age twenty you have had over 20,000 meals. If during the past two decades you have been eating too many of the wrong foods, then you are either overweight or unhealthy or well on your way to being there.

☐ In a previous book, LIVE LONGER NOW—THE FIRST ONE HUNDRED YEARS OF YOUR LIFE, I and my co-authors gave a detailed explanation of the main problem and what to do about it. Let me summarize some of the features from that work.

☐ The average American's diet consists of foods containing 40 to 45 percent of total calories in fat. It is no wonder that most Americans are overweight when you figure that one unit of fat has two and a half times more calories than either of the other food constituents: carbohydrates or protein.

☐ For example, let us assume that you are a fairly typical American eater and that you are consuming 2400 calories daily. This means that approximately 1100 of those calories are coming from the fat content of the foods you are eating. The number of calories, of course, varies depending on many factors including age, body weight, basal metabolism, and activity level. Too much fat, along with simple carbohydrates (simple sugars) and salt, leads to all sorts of degenerative diseases and other ailments.

☐ You can do a lot to improve your well-being just by cutting down on fatty foods in your daily diet. This not only will reduce your intake of one of the most detrimental food elements, but it will also help you to lose weight. And once the weight is gone, your body will tend to stabilize at its natural profile. If you want to stay healthy, cut down on fatty foods (fatty meats and dairy products, excess oils and deep-fried foods), simple carbo-hydrates (table sugar, candy, cookies, cake, pastries, soft drinks) and salty foods (table salt and any food products containing excessive amounts of salt). Eat all the fruit, vegetables, juices, lean meat, fish, poultry and grains you want. You will find it difficult to gain weight once you cut down on fatty foods. A side benefit is that your grocery bill will drop significantly. If you want the whole story, then I suggest you read LIVE LONGER NOW.

Note: LIVE LONGER NOW presents a dietary program for promoting good health. To follow this program 100 percent from the beginning may be too rigorous for some people. Therefore, you may want to gradually reduce the fats, sugars and salts in your diet rather than eliminate them suddenly.

☐ In addition to diet, frequent massage aids in breaking down fat and cellulite (merely another name for fat deposits) in your body.

☐ Another long-term benefit of massage is better skin and muscle tone, which aids in weight control.

EXERCISE Better to hunt in fields, for health unbought
Than fee the doctor for a nauseous draught.
The wise, for cure, on exercise depend;
God never made his work for man to mend.
John Dryden

Health is the vital principal of bliss
And exercise, of health.
James Thompson

Exercise is another important element in health and happiness. It helps drain off tension, keeps the body firm and trim, and strengthens internal organs. The best forms of exercise are the ones that cause your heart and lungs to get a sustained but not overloaded workout. Recommended exercises are running, jogging, roving, hiking, walking, swimming and riding a bicycle. But any form of exercise is better than none at all.
☐ If you are out of shape, start slowly and build up gradually. And cap your exercise sessions (after waiting at least one hour) with a soothing massage.

SEX No longer will sex be accepted as a thing apart, an isolated entity, a sexist privilege or an exploitable commodity. With each individual assuming responsibility for himself or herself alone, sex finally will be returned to the only position from which it can be viewed with comfort, and experienced with reliable fulfillment—that of a natural function.
Masters and Johnson

MASSAGE enhances sex; SEX enhances massage. In-

212

stead of being a vicious circle as are so many things in life, sex and massage can be thought of as a friendly circle.

☐ One of the best books available on sex is THE JOY OF SEX by Dr. Alex Comfort. The book is straight-forward, in good taste and beautifully illustrated.

☐ If you really get into massage, it will definitely improve your sex life. Since sex is a private matter, all I want to say to you is EACH TO HIS OR HER OWN and TOO MUCH WON'T HURT YOU.

MEDITATION

A man should combine his daily life
with the practice of meditation. This
very world of his, afflicted with the
threefold misery, would be transmuted
into a paradise.

                    Muktananda

Meditation is an increasingly popular and excellent way of centering and calming yourself.

☐ Get into a comfortable position where you will be free from all distractions for at least 15 minutes. Now close your eyes. Shove everything out of your mind. Breathe deeply. Let all the tension and worry melt away from your mind and body. Feel your muscles become rubbery.

☐ Simply repeat the sounds UUMM MAAW or SU over and over again. Keep repeating the sounds, especially if your attention begins to wander. You may use any man-tras (sounds) that feel good to you. I believe that medita-tion is something you can learn to do yourself. If, however, motivation is a problem, then I suggest you join the Transcendental Meditation Society—the $125 fee should keep you in the meditation groove.

☐ With some practice you should be able to meditate while riding in a vehicle (not when you're the driver, of course) on a break at work or practically any place where you can have a few undisturbed minutes to yourself.

YOGA Returning is the motion of the Tao
Yielding is the way of the Tao.
The ten thousand things are born of being.
Being is born of not being.

Lao Tsu

Yoga is an excellent way to keep your mind, body and joints supple and flexible. I could say a lot about yoga, but instead, I suggest you read the book PRACTICAL YOGA by Masahiro Oki. This is one of the most useful books on yoga available. You probably won't be able to do any of the exercises perfectly at first, but continued effort will soon pay off.

BREATHING A thing of beauty is a joy forever:
Its loveliness increases; it will never
Pass into nothingness; but still will keep
A bower quiet for us, and a sleep
Full of sweet dreams, and health, and quiet breathing.

John Keats

Shallow breathing occurs when stress is present. Deep breathing helps the relaxation process and builds up red blood cells.
☐ Learn to breathe deeply by taking in a deep breath

214

through your nose. Let it go around the roof of your mouth, then let it descend to the bottom of your abdomen.

☐ Now visualize the area from the bottom of your stomach to the top of your chest as a large glass vessel that you are going to fill with pure crystal-blue air, starting from the bottom. As you inhale, fill the lower half of the vessel with air and progress up to the top of your shoulders. Hold your breath for a count of three, and then slowly let all the air out through your mouth.

☐ When you think all the air is out, give a final HUUUGGGH to expel that remaining pocket of air. You will automatically start the process over again.

☐ Deep breathing is a good tonic any time you feel tension building up.

All day, the same our postures were,
And we said nothing, all the day.
     John Donne

POSTURE

Prolonged tenseness can result in a slumped posture.

☐ You probably heard "Stand up straight" or something similar when you were a child. Maybe one of the reasons you slumped was that you and your parents were out of touch with each other.

☐ Poor posture results in low back pain. This is a commonplace physical ailment. If not corrected, it can result in a permanent defect. Massage, along with exercise, yoga and keeping the shoulders and spine erect, can aid in correcting this modern-day back malady.

☐ Practice sitting and standing up straight. Imagine a

cord is tied to the top of your head. Now visualize some-one pulling upward on the cord just to the point where you would begin to feel your body lift off the chair or floor.

☐ The Japanese are masters at transistorizing and com-pacting things. And they have reduced the number of posture exercises into a 5-minute daily experience. Read the book MAKKŌ-HŌ—FIVE MINUTES' PHYSICAL FITNESS by Haruka Nagai. With enough practice, good posture will become second nature.

☐ Whatever you get into, whether it be a different form of massage, exercise, diet, yoga or meditation, take it one step at a time. Give each method a chance and don't overdo anything.

If the Tasadays, remnants of a stone age culture recently discovered in the Philippines, are an example of primitive communication, perhaps their constant use of warm, enfolding embraces and their loving touches should make us think more deeply about the communication power of the skin. The Tasadays have no words for weapons or war or hate. Has the natural love and wonder of man been disserviced by unnatural concepts of human behavior for so long that we have forgotten that skin communication once led to peace and understanding?

Barbara B. Brown
NEW MIND, NOW BODY

SUGGESTED READING

I have listed below some worthwhile books that I place in the category of "improving the human condition."

☐ Buscaglia, Leo F., LOVE. Thorofare: Charles B. Slack Publications, 1973.

☐ Davis, Flora, INSIDE INTUITION: WHAT WE KNOW ABOUT NONVERBAL COMMUNICATION. New York: McGraw-Hill, Inc., 1973.

☐ Gunther, Bernard, SENSE RELAXATION BELOW YOUR MIND. New York: Macmillan, Inc., 1968.

☐ Montagu, Ashley, TOUCHING: THE HUMAN SIGNIFICANCE OF THE SKIN. New York: Columbia University Press, 1971.

☐ Morris, Desmond, INTIMATE BEHAVIOUR. New York: Random House, Inc., 1972.

☐ Nance, John, THE GENTLE TASADAY. New York: Harcourt, Brace, Jovanovitch, 1975.

TOUCHING, NONVERBAL COMMUNICATION AND BODY LANGUAGE

☐ Comfort, Alex, THE JOY OF SEX. New York: Crown Publishers, Inc., 1972.

☐ ————, MORE JOY. New York: Simon & Schuster, Inc., 1975.

☐ Lowen, Alexander, PLEASURE: A CREATIVE APPROACH TO LIFE. New York: Penguin Books, Inc., 1975.

☐ Masters, William H. and Johnson, Virginia E., THE PLEASURE BOND: A NEW LOOK AT SEXUALITY AND COMMITMENT. Boston: Little, Brown and Company, 1975.

SEXUAL PLEASURE

STRESS AND NERVOUS TENSION

- [ ] Bloomfield, Harold H., Cain, Michael Peter, and Jaffe, Denny T., TM: DISCOVERING INNER ENERGY AND OVERCOMING STRESS. New York: Delacorte Press, 1975.
- [ ] Friedman, Meyer and Rosenman, Ray H., TYPE A BEHAVIOR AND YOUR HEART. New York: Alfred A. Knopf, Inc., 1974.
- [ ] McQuade, Walter and Aikman, Ann, STRESS. New York: E. P. Dutton & Company, Inc., 1974.
- [ ] Newman, Mildred and Berkowitz, Bernard, HOW TO BE YOUR OWN BEST FRIEND. New York: Ballantine Books, Inc., 1974.
- [ ] Selye, Hans, THE STRESS OF LIFE. New York: McGraw-Hill, 1975.
- [ ] ———, STRESS WITHOUT DISTRESS. Philadelphia and New York: J. B. Lippincott Company, 1974.

HEALTH, NUTRITION, EATING AND EXERCISE

- [ ] Fox, Edward L. and Mathews, Donald K., INTERVAL TRAINING: CONDITIONING FOR SPORTS AND PHYSICAL FITNESS. Philadelphia: W. B. Saunders Company, 1974.
- [ ] Leonard, Jon; Hofer, Jack and Pritikin, Nathan, LIVE LONGER NOW: THE FIRST HUNDRED YEARS OF YOUR LIFE. New York: Grosset & Dunlap, Inc., 1974.
- [ ] Mayer, Jean, HEALTH. New York: Van Nostrand Reinhold Company, 1974.

CONTEMPLATION

- [ ] Dass, Ram, THE ONLY DANCE THERE IS. New York: Jason Aronson, Inc., 1974.
- [ ] English, Jane and Feng, Gia-Fu, TAO TE CHING. New York: Random House, Inc., 1972.
- [ ] Golas, Thaddeus, THE LAZY MAN'S GUIDE TO EN-LIGHTENMENT. Seed Center, 1972.
- [ ] Suzuki, Shunryu, ZEN MIND, BEGINNER'S MIND. New York: John Weatherhill, Inc., 1970.
- [ ] Watts, Alan, THE BOOK: ON THE TABOO AGAINST KNOWING WHO YOU ARE. New York: Random House, Inc., 1972.
- [ ] ———, THIS IS IT AND OTHER ESSAYS ON ZEN AND SPIRITUAL EXPERIENCES. New York: Pantheon Books, Inc., 1960.

INDEX

ACKNOWLEDGMENTS

Warm and soothing acknowledgments to:
  Marjett Schille, for her superb illustrations;
  Patty Siedlak, for her skillful photography which
    Marjett illustrated;
  The Old Man of the Beach who told me "The Tale of
    the Loving Hands."
Other bodily helpers, believers and supporters:
  Gretchen, Michael, Bob, Dave, Judy, Beverly, Wally,
    Jeanne, Anita, Nelleke, Allan, Lorraine, Myrna.

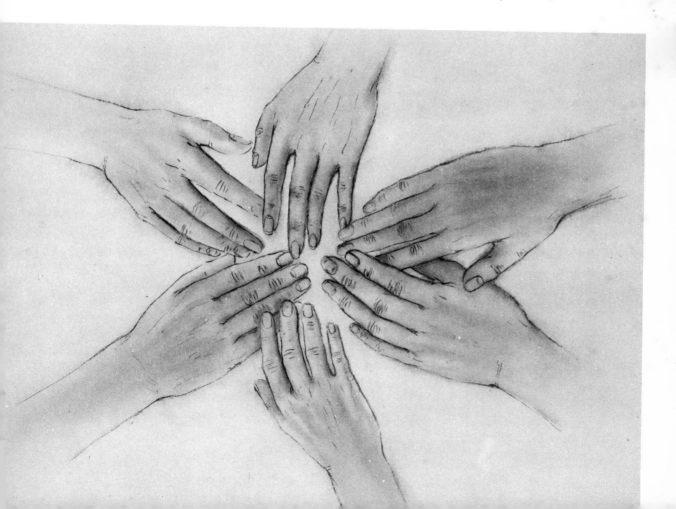